AF715743

SPARK

A PHYSICIAN'S PATH TO PURPOSE

DIMITRI TITO

Copyright © 2025 by Dimitri Tito

All rights reserved.

No part of this book may be reproduced in any form or by any electronic or mechanical means, including information storage and retrieval systems, without written permission from the author, except for the use of brief quotations in a book review.

Cover Design: L. Douglas Hogan

CONTENTS

IN LOVING MEMORY OF...

Maman Magni Tadjou Lydie
Maman Kamga Tabie
Papa Kamga Wouemgnie Emmanuel

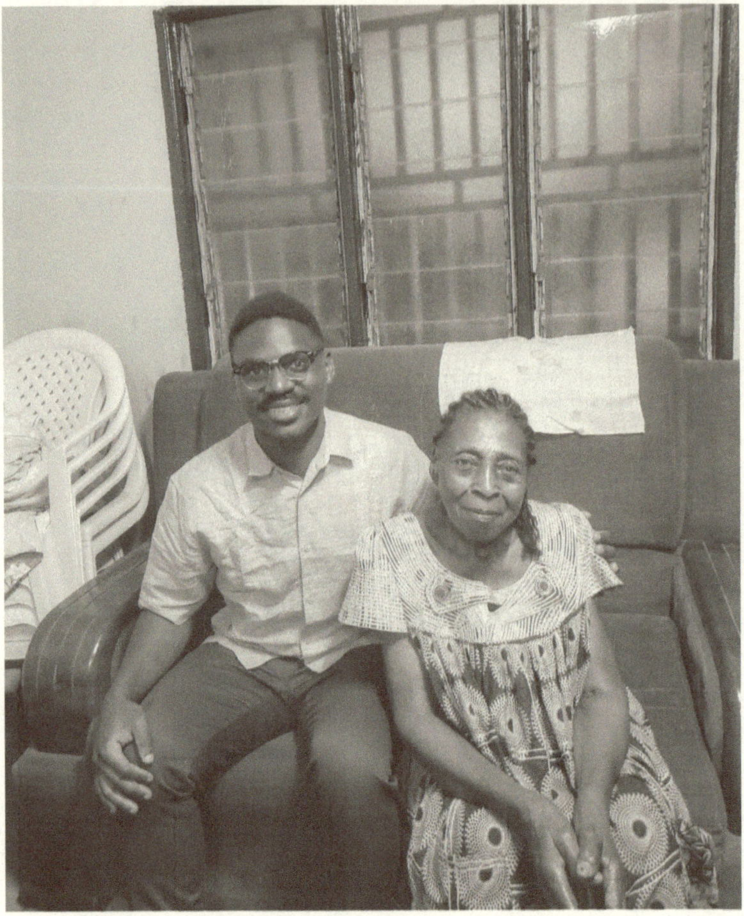

This book is dedicated to the memory of my beloved grandmother, Maman Magne. Her life as a merchant was a testament to strength and wisdom, and the skills she imparted to me have been an enduring source of inspiration. Though she is no longer with us, the connection we shared and the values she instilled continue to guide me on this physician's journey to purpose.

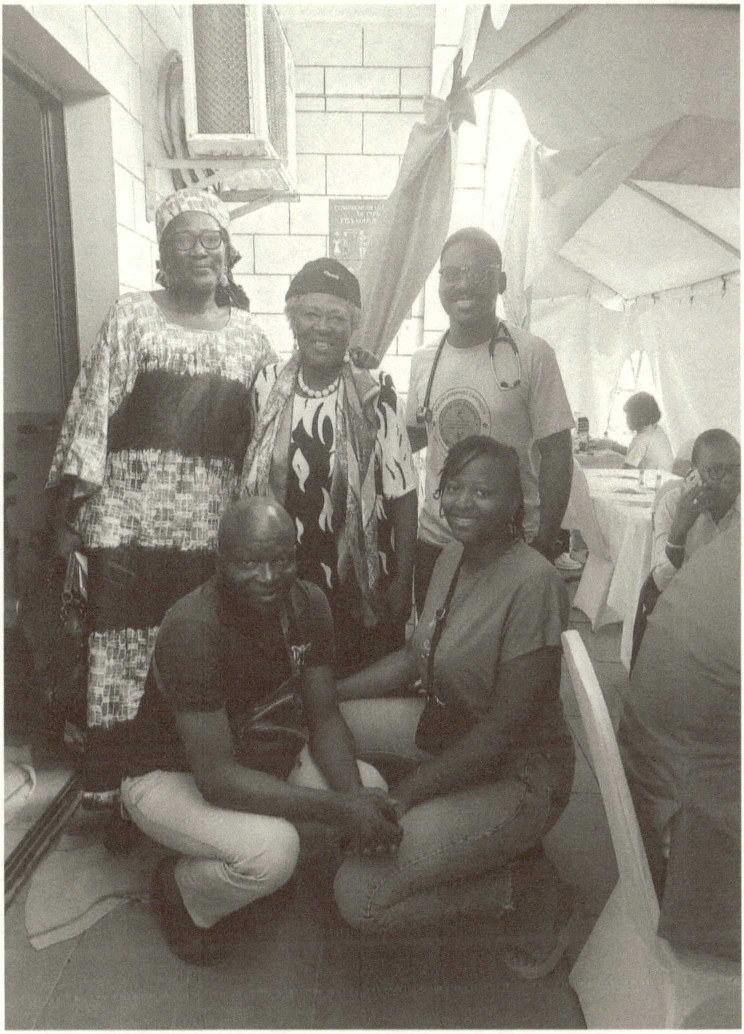

To my grandmother-in-law (center), a remarkable woman of God, whose presence in this picture is a reminder of her enduring legacy. She passed away two months before my wedding, leaving a void, but also an inheritance of faith and grace that continues to inspire. This book is a tribute to her spirit and the values she embodied, which are integral to my own journey as a physician seeking to live a life of purpose.

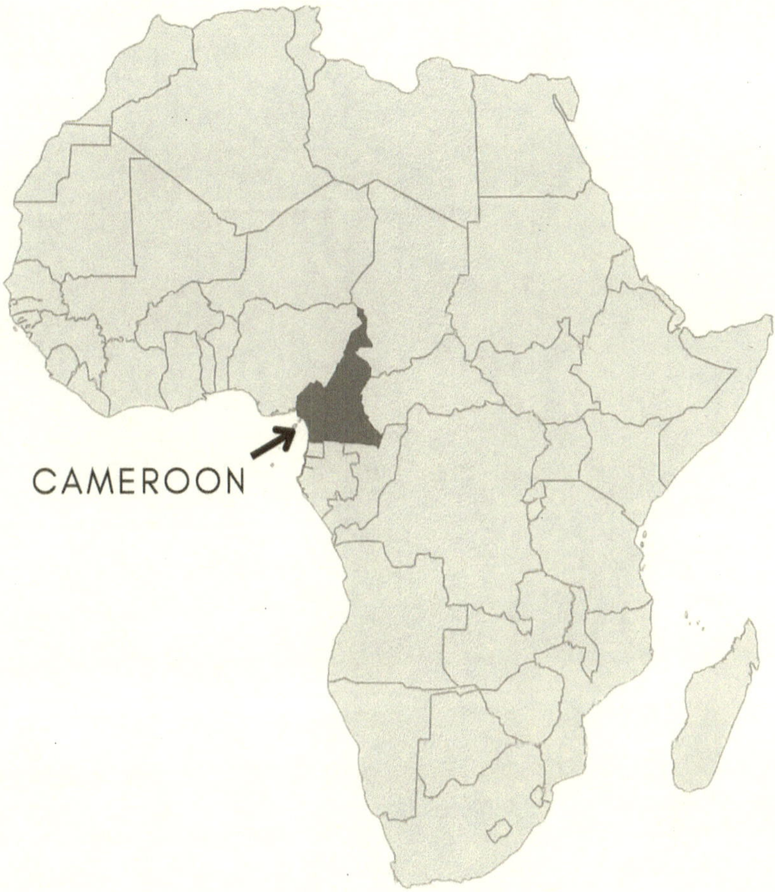
CAMEROON

AUTHOR'S NOTE

This book is both a continuation and an evolution.

When I first wrote *A Fire in Appalachia*, I shared the journey of a young man from humble beginnings—one who dared to pursue medicine with heart, grit, and an unshakable belief in service. That story reflected where I was then: fresh from the trenches of medical school, still feeling the fire of every challenge, every lesson, every patient who changed me. It was raw, urgent, and honest.

But time moves forward, and so do we.

Spark: A Physician's Path to Purpose is my way of revisiting that story—not to retell it, but to deepen it. I've taken parts of *A Fire in Appalachia* and rewritten them with the clarity that only hindsight can offer. I've also added new chapters that bring you up to date with where I am now—both professionally and personally. This isn't just an update. It's an expansion of the themes that matter most to me: purpose, resilience, identity, and the responsibility we all carry to be of use in this world.

If you've read my first book, you'll recognize familiar moments, now shaped with broader reflection. If this is your first time picking up my story, welcome. I hope it lights something in you.

Thank you for walking this path with me.

- Dimi Tito

INTRODUCTION

My name is Emmanuel Dimitri Foko Tito but you can call me Dimi, and I was born in Douala, Cameroon—the wealthiest place on Earth. That might surprise you. What came to mind when you read the word *Cameroon*? Be honest. There's no judgment here. Whatever you imagined, you're likely not alone.

If you're like many people from what is often called the "developed world," the images that filled your mind may have been shaped long ago: maybe malnourished children with hollow eyes and bloated stomachs; perhaps fierce, painted warriors adorned in feathers and bones, screaming war cries into the sky; or wandering nomads in a sun-scorched desert, chasing mirages and praying to ancient gods for water. Maybe, you just pictured poverty. Deep, relentless poverty.

You'd be wrong—but you wouldn't be alone.

When I first came to the United States, I encountered many people who imagined my country in exactly those ways. At first, I was offended. How could they see my home through such a narrow lens? But over time, I came to understand: it wasn't really their fault. From childhood, they'd been fed these images—by Hollywood movies set in "Africa," by charity ads and mission trips, by school textbooks that glossed over everything but hardship. Maybe even from a milk carton in the cafeteria bearing the haunted face of a skeletal child.

And so, if Cameroon is in Africa, and Africa is all those things, then surely Cameroon must be too. Right?

Yes, Cameroon is in Africa. And no, it doesn't have the material wealth of countries labeled "first world." Like every nation, it has its share of struggles—we'll talk about those in this book. But Cameroon is *not* poor. Not in the way most people think.

Cameroon holds a kind of wealth that no hardship can diminish. It is a nation of millions bound together by something far greater than money: *family*. And there is nothing more valuable than that.

But family is a choice. Always. In life, we decide what kind of people we will be. We can choose to hoard what we have, or we can choose to share. We can look away from others' pain—or we can lift them up. We can live for ourselves, or we can live for something bigger. From my earliest memories, I've been surrounded by people who chose the latter. People who gave, who loved, who served, who made their lives about others. Because of them, even though I was born into a country facing economic hardship, I never once felt poor. I lived in the wealth of community, of compassion, of connection. I was rich in every way that mattered.

My name is Dimi—but some know me as Square Root, or Sena, or Posterchild. We'll get to that later.

I was born in Kotto, a crowded residential district on the edge of Douala, Cameroon's economic heart in Central Africa. It was 1994. That year, the average annual income in Cameroon was just $1,600. We were ranked the 26th poorest country on what is often called the poorest continent on Earth. And yet, if you had asked me—or my siblings, or my parents, or our neighbors—we all would have told you the same thing: *We had plenty.*

In time, I would travel to the United States, learn English, study Biomedical Engineering and later Medicine. I would be given the incredible opportunity to help others the same way I had always been helped: by giving what I have, and doing it with love.

This is the story I want to tell you.

It's not a story of dramatic adversity or heroic comeback. Those stories are important, and many people have lived them—but they are not mine.

Mine is a simpler story. A story of how a life, no matter how humble its beginnings, can become something extraordinary—not by chasing greatness for its own sake, but by choosing to serve, to love, to remember. A story about how far someone can go when they carry with them the lessons of their youth. A story about generosity, inspiration, and community. A story about becoming part of something bigger than yourself.

This is the story of how a single spark, when protected and nourished, can grow into a powerful flame.

1

MERCY

DOUALA WAS the first world I knew—a humid, breathing city that smelled of rain on hot asphalt and the salt of the nearby sea. I lived there with my family until I was sixteen, in a household that was small by Cameroonian standards: just five children. Landry and Wilfried, my older brothers, came first. I was the middle child, trailed by Jordan, then Nora, the youngest and only daughter, whose spotless record —never once in trouble—was something of a family marvel.

Our father was Emmanuel, as was his father before him, and all of us boys carried the name as well. It was a family thread, binding us in name, though we moved through life under our middle names or softened nicknames. That is how I came to be Dimi. Our mother, Isabelle, was the quiet anchor who kept us all from drifting too far from home.

We were seven beneath our roof, but the boundaries of family stretched beyond concrete walls. It spilled into the grid of our neighborhood—into the narrow streets, the shaded alleys, the foot-worn paths that threaded between houses. Neighbors were aunts and uncles in all but blood. Friends were brothers and sisters.

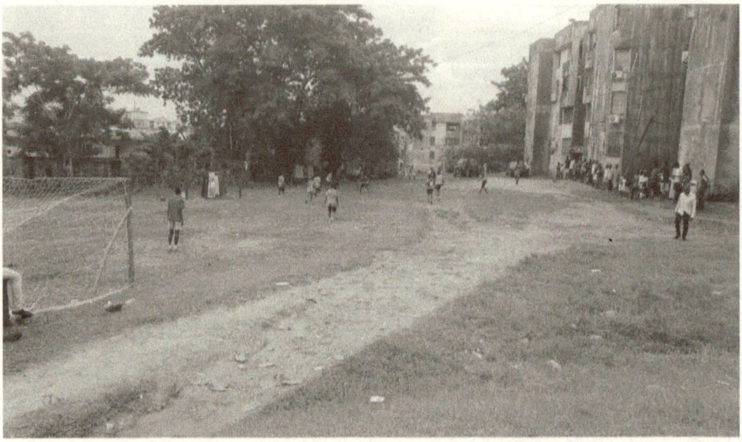

The heart of my beginnings, the field where dreams first took flight. This is my neighborhood in Kotto, Douala, Cameroon, the vibrant place where I grew up, spending countless hours playing soccer on this very field. More than just a playground, it was a classroom of life, teaching me teamwork, resilience, and the joy of pursuing a shared goal. This image is a powerful reminder of my roots, the simple pleasures that shaped my character, and the enduring connection to the place I proudly call home.

Douala, like so many of Africa's great cities, bore the bones of another time. The colonial empires that had once claimed it left behind their roads, their drainage channels, their grand ambitions—all of it weathered and patched, never quite keeping pace with the present. The main arteries of the city reached outward, paved in mismatched asphalt, leading to the countryside. Beyond them, the streets were fractured, some surrendered to dust and dirt, others never paved at all. When the rains came, water pooled and wandered, cutting its own paths as it had long before concrete arrived.

Buildings leaned into each other, shoulder to shoulder. They were not ancient, but they looked tired—structures made to serve one purpose, now repurposed again and again, patched over like old wounds. Few rose higher than four stories; a handful scraped at ten. The air between them was thin, filled with the noise of traffic and voices and the hum of generators.

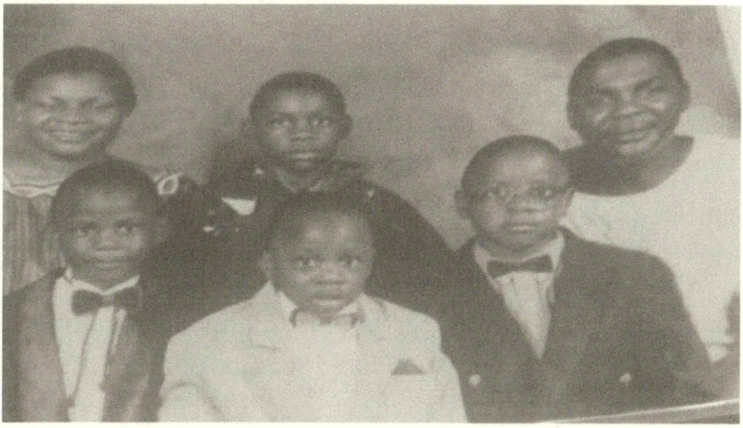

The pillars of my strength, the source of my inspiration. My parents and siblings – three brothers and one sister – captured in a moment of togetherness. This image represents the unwavering support, guidance, and love that have shaped my journey and continue to ground me. They are the reason I strive for purpose and the reminder of what truly matters.From left to right, Isabelle (mother), Landry (oldest brother), Dimi (myself), Jordan (younger brother), Wilfried (older brother), Emmanuel (Father).

I grew up in Kotto, in the northwest of the city, in a pocket village of about thirty homes. Douala was full of such clusters—rows of whitewashed concrete houses arranged like puzzle pieces around a shared space, most often a soccer field. The roofs were flat, the walls straight, and the shapes boxy, as though someone had built them from stacked blocks. Fences enclosed backyards where we children spent our days, shouting over the drone of cicadas, the sound bouncing from wall to wall.

Some families built their homes with their own hands. Others, like ours, bought government-built houses and shaped them into something personal. My father's work made that possible. His shop sold whatever he thought the city might want: radios and shirts, shoes and bags, and later, filtered water. The water came in bottles, or in small plastic bags you could tear open with your teeth or pierce with a straw. He was always looking for the next thing to add to his shelves, but not out of greed. For him, success was a tide that lifted the whole shore—our family, our neighbors, anyone within reach.

My mother kept a smaller store, one lined with dresses and shirts that swayed when the fan turned. She had no interest in expansion. Her work was here, at home, making sure our lives ran smoothly, making sure we studied. She was the one who noticed if we were straying, the one who pulled us back. But that's a story for later.

Between my parents' two businesses and their tireless effort, we lived comfortably by Cameroonian standards, though "middle-class" was not a term often spoken there. Our home was not grand, but it was ours, and every space within it carried the imprint of our lives.

From the street, you'd first see the white front wall, broken by two red gates—one small, one large. The smaller gate opened to the front door; the larger swung wide enough for a car to pass through. Yes, we had two, parked one behind the other in what we called the garage, though the word might conjure the wrong image for an American reader. There was no door, no automatic hum of a motorized opener, no climate control—just a broad opening in the wall, its floor a scatter of crushed stone and whatever grass dared to grow there.

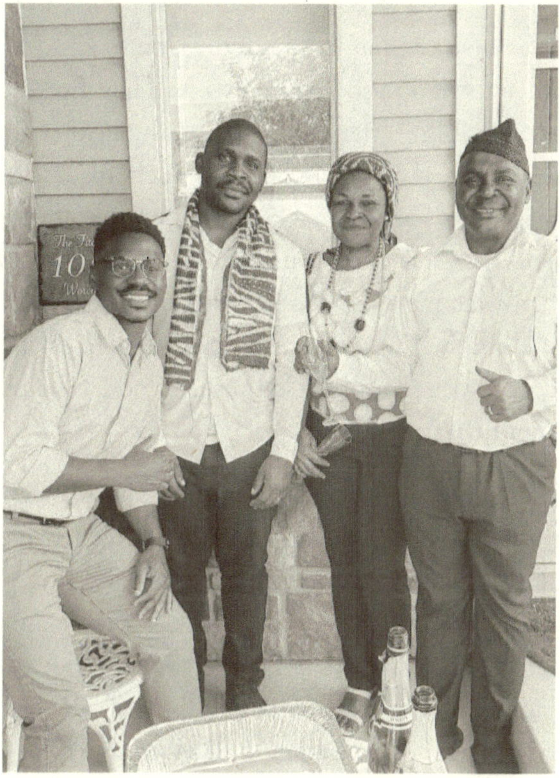

In this cherished moment, surrounded by my dearest parents and eldest brother, Landry Tito, celebrating a new beginning at my nephew's baptism. This image reminds me of the foundational love and unwavering support that have always been my anchor, fueling my journey toward purpose.

From the garage, you stepped directly into the first kitchen—the dining kitchen. Here we served and ate our meals. There was a sink, cupboards, and counters, but no oven, no stove. In Cameroonian homes, cooking took place in a second, smaller kitchen, tucked away so that the sights and smells of preparation, and the clutter of dirty dishes, stayed hidden from the eyes of guests. Meals were meant to be enjoyed in calm and order; the chaos of cooking could wait until later.

Beyond the first kitchen lay the living room, and from there, doors and stairs led to the bedrooms. We had five in all. The youngest two siblings shared one room, the next two another. The eldest child always had a room to themselves—a small rite of passage in Cameroon—and my parents, of course, had their own. That left one room open, a guest room, which in our culture was more a necessity than a luxury. If someone came for dinner, it was common for them to stay the night. After all, they were family, whether by blood or by bond, and you did not turn family away.

The walls inside were mostly painted concrete, some lined with brightly colored ceramic tiles in patterned borders or full panels. The decorations spoke of who we were: wooden shelves holding carved figures, masks with painted eyes, tanned animal skins stretched like tapestries. Between them hung framed Bible verses—reminders of the faith that anchored our lives. Cameroon is a deeply religious country, and our family was no exception. All the Emmanuels in our home carried the name that means *God is with us*—a truth we believed and displayed.

There were no carpets. The floors were tile or polished wood, cool under bare feet and easy to sweep clean. Our bedrooms were small—just enough space for a bed or bunk, a narrow walking path, and shelves lining the walls. I never thought them cramped until I came to America, where even the smallest apartments seemed sprawling by comparison. In

Douala, our rooms had always felt right-sized—nothing wasted, nothing missing.

To someone reading this from a place of abundance, our way of living might seem modest, even sparse, as though our lives were measured in what we lacked. But that is not the truth of it. In Cameroon, life is measured in connection—in the network of family and neighbors who take care of one another. However little you have, it is enough, because it is shared. If we needed sugar, we went next door and asked. If a neighbor needed an axe, they came to us. You gave without keeping tally, and you received without debt.

In our neighborhood, everyone knew everyone, which meant there were always eyes on the street. Children roamed far from their own yards without fear, because every adult was their guardian. The sound of laughter carried down the alleyways, and if a ball rolled into a stranger's yard, it came back without question. This was the unspoken covenant of our lives: we were all family, and in a family, no one is truly alone.

In Cameroon, warmth is the default setting. Encounters begin with a wave, a smile, and a question that reaches beyond the moment—about your day, your father's business, or whether your sister has recovered from her cold. These exchanges are not small talk; they are acknowledgments that your life is seen, remembered. Unlike in America, where eye contact is often avoided and time with friends scheduled into neat calendar squares, we lived in a place where connection required no appointment.

If you were headed to the soccer field, you didn't call ahead or send a message—you knocked on the doors of the kids you wanted to join you. They came, or they didn't. Most of the time, they did. If you wanted to see a friend, you simply went to their house, leaned your head through the doorway, and called their name. Chances were, they were already there, ready to welcome you inside for the day. And if they weren't, their parents would wave you in, offer a seat, and before long, a plate of food.

That, too, was part of our wealth. In Cameroon, every adult is a guardian, every home a second home. I spent entire days at friends' houses, often alongside other neighborhood children. At mealtimes, no one was sent away. Pots were filled with enough for everyone. Feeding someone else's child was an honor, not a burden, and for those hours you were not a guest—you were one of theirs. If you were hungry, they fed you. If you had a problem, they helped you solve it. If you misbehaved, they punished you without hesitation, and your own parents would expect no less. In our house, we did the same.

I knew a fair bit about being punished. I wasn't a bad kid, just... accident-prone. A soccer ball through a window, a plate slipping from my hands, a glass tipped into the wrong lap—my disasters were small but frequent. For a stretch of time, my siblings and friends wouldn't even let me touch the video game console or television for fear I'd break them. My reputation for clumsiness was so well-earned that, some days, they kept their distance entirely.

Still, home was where we all returned when the day wound down—unless we were sleeping at a friend's. My parents worked from morning until late in the evening, often arriving around nine. When we heard the horn at the gate, it was the oldest child's job to open it so they could drive in—a small act, but one heavy with respect. We waited for them eagerly. My father would go straight to the living room, and we would gather around him, spilling our stories of the day, listening to his in turn. He never missed the chance to fold a lesson into his words, to praise or correct us according to the quiet codes of our culture.

My mother, after showering, would head to the kitchen to prepare dinner, which we often ate around ten at night. I never thought that unusual until I moved to the United States, where the last meal of the day is served hours earlier. For us, dinner was a shared event, and no one began eating until everyone was seated. It was a rule woven into the fabric of our lives, one mirrored in many homes across the city.

We children, of course, found our own ways to keep ourselves fed during the day—snacks from neighbors, small purchases from street vendors, bowls of fruit plucked from trees along the paths. We never went hungry.

After dinner, my mother became our teacher. She had once dreamed of being one, though life had steered her elsewhere. Even so, she carried that skill in her bones. Tutoring us in our studies seemed to light something in her, even when we groaned over the work. For her, it was not just about homework—it was about shaping us into capable people. And in that, she was relentless.

Life in Cameroon was like this for most: hard work, shared resources, enough for everyone. It was not a life of excess, but of abundance measured in connection, care, and the certainty that you belonged somewhere.

Yet life in Cameroon, for all its connection and generosity, is not without its shadows. Gratitude can soften the edges, but it does not erase the hard lines of reality. There are challenges—some woven deep into the fabric of our society—that cannot be ignored. One of the most pressing is the uneven access to modern, consistent, high-quality medical care.

In Cameroon, those who tend to the sick fall into two broad groups: doctors and traditional healers. Doctors are much like their counterparts in wealthier nations—educated, formally trained, grounded in the science of modern medicine. They work with needles and pills, scalpels and stethoscopes. Traditional healers, by contrast, draw on the accumulated knowledge of generations, handed down through family lines and cultural memory. They use herbs, poultices, and tinctures mixed with mortar and pestle, their cures rooted as much in ritual as in remedy.

An outsider might wonder why Cameroonians, faced with illness, wouldn't simply bypass the healer and go straight to the doctor. On paper, it seems obvious. But reality here is not written in the clean lines of logic—it is shaped by scarcity. The truth is, while our doctors are skilled and devoted, there are far too few of them for the people they serve. Clinics are overburdened, resources stretched thin.

To see a doctor, you may wait weeks. And when your turn comes, there is no guarantee the clinic will have what you need—especially if your illness demands more than basic care. An X-ray machine might be broken, an MRI might be hours away in another city, a CT scanner might not exist in your province at all.

It's often said that cancer rates are lower here than in the developed world. I want to believe that is true. But a quiet question always lingers: how many cases simply go undiagnosed? In terms of medical infrastructure, Cameroon is undeniably poor. Still, the picture is not as desperate as some imagine.

Traditional healers remain more numerous than doctors, and for many ailments—particularly those not considered life-threatening—they are the first stop. If you have the flu, a stubborn stomach bug, or a fever without cause, you may visit your neighborhood healer. They will examine you with the practiced eye of someone steeped in their craft, name your illness, and prescribe a remedy—a bitter tea, a paste to spread across your skin, a packet of leaves to boil and inhale.

It's important to understand that healers in Cameroon are not shadowy mystics hidden away in smoke-filled rooms. They are respected professionals whose craft is rooted in deep cultural tradition. In many cases, they ease the discomfort of everyday illnesses, offering relief when the ailment is more nuisance than threat. Their role has been vital for centuries, not only here but across countless ancient cultures.

What is remarkable—perhaps surprising to outsiders—is the harmony between doctors and healers in Cameroon. They are not rivals but partners of a sort, working along the same chain of care. A patient might first visit a healer for diagnosis and treatment, and if the illness lingers or proves more serious than expected, the healer will often urge them to see a doctor. In turn, doctors will reach out to the healer to learn what they have already tried—the remedies given, the symptoms observed, the patient's history.

Though they may work in separate spaces—one in a clinic, the other in a courtyard or small room—the healer acts as an informal extension of the doctor's staff. And when the doctor's work is done, the patient often returns to the healer for follow-up care, for prescriptions, for the comfort of a familiar hand. It is not a perfect system, but in a place where resources are few, it is one that holds genuine value.

Still, even with such cooperation, the limits are stark. Cameroon carries the weight of diseases that never loosen their grip—malaria, cholera, tuberculosis, yellow fever. When these illnesses flare, the strain on local doctors is immense, and often the expertise or equipment needed is simply not there. In this gap, the healer's role can sometimes outpace that of the physician, relying on time-worn remedies when modern solutions are out of reach.

It was in this landscape of scarcity that I first encountered a very different kind of care—one that arrived not from within Cameroon but from far beyond its shores. I was nine years old when I first heard of Mercy Ships, though in truth, they had been coming to Douala for years. Their arrival was always an event—advertisements posted on walls and lampposts, voices on the radio, segments on the evening news announcing that they would be in port through August and September. But this was the first year I needed them. In fact, I would need them twice.

When Mercy Ships comes, the city hums with anticipation. Their great white vessel docks at the busy port, a floating hospital that draws people from every corner of the country.

Some come with small complaints—a cough that won't leave, a persistent fever. Others arrive with conditions so grave that hope has worn thin: tumors, advanced infections, illnesses that local medicine has no answer for. But no one is turned away. Whether the problem is a common cold or an inoperable cancer, Mercy Ships offers care with the same quiet compassion.

And for those who cannot afford treatment anywhere else, there is an even greater gift: it is free. At most, the cost is so minimal that even families of modest means can pay. But the generosity extends further. Mercy Ships brings not only doctors and nurses but supplies—thermometers, bandages, antiseptics, vitamins, and countless other necessities. They train local practitioners, equipping them with new skills, new techniques. They hold public workshops so that ordinary people can learn to better care for themselves and their families. Parents often send their children, who return with care packages full of essentials, their small hands gripping treasures that will keep a household healthy through the season.

For me, that first visit to Mercy Ships was unforgettable—not only because of the treatment I received, but because it revealed a truth I had never fully understood: that kindness can sail across oceans, dock in a city, and change the lives of people it has never met.

Every day during the one or two months the Mercy Ships are anchored at port, the lines began before sunrise. People arrived by any means they could—on foot, by bus, clinging to the sides of crowded taxis, or in the backs of trucks. Some walked for hours, even days, to reach Douala. My family was fortunate; when it was our turn, we drove from Kotto. My ailments each time I visited made walking the several-hour distance impossible.

The first visit was for a broken foot I had earned on the soccer field. We left while the sky was still blue-black, the air heavy with the scent of dew, and by the time we reached the port, the horizon was just beginning to blush with light. Even at that hour, the line curved like a slow-moving river along the dock.

But no one complained. In that line, gratitude outweighed discomfort. Every person there knew the wait would be worth it, that at the end of it stood care unlike anything we could find elsewhere in the country.

Crossing onto the ship was like stepping into another world. The air inside was cool, the hallways gleaming white. The system was swift, precise. First came a full physical examination, then a nurse who listened carefully—watching as much as hearing—before you were ushered to a doctor who would guide your treatment from that moment forward. Most of the staff spoke English; most of us did not. If you were lucky, you found a nurse fluent in French, or someone who could translate. But even without words, they understood you. They read pain in your posture, illness in the way you held yourself.

For my foot, the process was smooth. X-rays revealed a clean break in one of my metatarsals. They splinted it properly, fitted me with a brand-new crutch, handed me a bag of medical supplies, and sent me home with careful instructions for recovery. My foot healed quickly, and I thought my time with the Mercy Ships for that year was over.

It wasn't.

A few weeks later, I caught what we believed was a stubborn cold. At first, it was nothing unusual—coughing, sneezing, a runny nose. My mother brewed the traditional remedy: hot water steeped with honey, ginger, and a blend of native herbs and spices. But instead of improving, my symptoms deepened. By the second week, new ones emerged—relentless diarrhea, dehydration no amount of water could quench, food that refused to stay down, and fevers spiking as high as 105 degrees.

We decided it was the flu, the kind that required more than home remedies, and returned to the Mercy Ships. That morning, standing in the line again, every joint throbbed, my muscles shuddered beneath my skin, and it took all my effort to stay upright. But I was still hopeful. I believed—knew—that I was about to receive the best care possible for my illness.

When the doctors examined me, they wasted no time in telling us the truth: it wasn't the flu. It was malaria. They moved quickly, starting IV fluids and antibiotics that stayed in my arm for the rest of the day. When they sent me home, it was with a month's supply of medication and instructions for every dose. My appetite returned almost immediately. Within a week, my strength had followed, and by the second, I was whole again.

It wouldn't be my last visit. Over the years, I would return to the ships many times—three of those for malaria. Other visits were for the free medical supplies, or simply to walk their bright corridors. They even had a library on board, and I spent hours there, running my fingers over spines, pulling books from shelves, disappearing into worlds far beyond the port city.

But what stayed with me most was not the medicine, nor even the cures—it was the people. The doctors and nurses who had left their own practices, their own countries, to serve strangers in need. Men and women who, for a season, made our struggles their own. As a child, I could not fully understand the weight of that generosity. But I felt it. I felt it in the way they looked at me, in the way their hands worked carefully over my injuries, in the way they made me feel seen, even in my smallest and weakest moments.

And that feeling—the knowledge that someone who had more than you could choose to give without asking for anything in return—never left me.

2

FROM SQUARE ROOT TO SENA

Growing up, I loved school—not so much the hours spent in a classroom at first, but the journey to get there and the walk back home. In Cameroon, movement itself felt like freedom. Getting around was different from what most children in the developed world experience. As I've mentioned before, children were trusted to roam on their own from an early age. It wasn't because crime didn't exist—of course it did—but it rarely touched us. The kind of violence I would later learn to associate with children—kidnappings, abductions, even school shootings—simply wasn't part of our lives. Crime in Cameroon was aimed elsewhere: at the wealthy, at businesses, at banks, and most often under cover of night in the commercial districts. For us, the streets were safe.

And so, even though school was an hour's walk from my house, I made the trip on foot every day. That walk became the highlight of my childhood, a ritual stitched into my memory more vividly than most classroom lessons. We neighborhood children built our own small systems of travel, meeting at certain points along the way, weaving routes that scattered us to different schools but always gave us companionship for part of the journey. Without phones, we relied on word of mouth and the plan made the day before—tomorrow we'll meet here, take this path, walk together until that crossing. By morning, we'd gather at the appointed place, and the adventure would begin.

School began at seven. Which meant that at five, my mother would already be stirring us awake, preparing breakfast in the dim glow before dawn. Breakfast in Cameroon was never light; it was the previous night's dinner reheated, something hearty to carry us through—couscous and sauce, or thick porridge, or fried plantains. Food was always filling, never delicate. By six, we were out the door, our small allowances tucked into our pockets—about 1,000 CFA for the week, enough to buy a snack or supplement a meal while we were gone. It sounds like plenty, but really it was just survival money, because once we left, we wouldn't see our parents again until late at night, sometimes nine o'clock or later.

By the time I was seven, I no longer needed my older siblings to guide me. I could navigate my own path, confident in the web of friends and meeting points along the way. I would set off alone from the gate, then turn down alleys, cut across patches of sandy road, and join the others. Our routes took us through a patchwork of city life: paved stretches that gave way to dirt tracks, crooked alleys, sudden bursts of greenery where wooded paths cut across neighborhoods.

And we never walked in silence. We made games out of the journey, teased one another, argued about movies or the latest soccer scores, swapped small secrets, sang until our voices carried across the fields. Singing was in our blood—traditional songs, folk rhythms, call-and-response chants passed down for generations. It was how we entertained ourselves, how we reminded each other of who we were. Those songs, those long walks through the waking streets of Douala, wove us together tighter than school ever did.

Vendors were always waiting along the routes, their carts parked at the busiest crossings where children passed in steady streams. From them we could buy roasted peanuts wrapped in paper, corn grilled over open coals, sticky caramels, or small cakes warm from the pan. Whatever one child bought, they shared—it was not a matter of generosity so much as simple culture. Food belonged to everyone.

I always bought something, though usually something small. I was careful with my coins. Beneath my bed, hidden in the shadows, I kept a little wooden safe with a narrow slot at the top—wide enough to slip money in, too narrow to slip your hand back out. Later, in the United States, I would learn such things were called piggy banks, shaped like fat little animals. Mine was only a box, plain and square, but it served the same purpose. Each week I saved what I could, and at year's end, I cracked it open and handed the contents to my parents, who used the money to buy me a new soccer ball or, if I was lucky, a video game.

But even with saving on my mind, I never walked empty-handed. I always bought something to share with the others—enough to keep the ritual alive. As we moved along, eating our snacks, the group would thin. Children peeled off in ones and twos, veering down the alleys toward their schools. By the time I reached mine, only a handful remained, sometimes just one or two. Those were the ones I grew closest to—not because we were bound by anything extraordinary, but because we had the longest stretch of road together. Over the years, as faces came and went, as schools changed, we adjusted our routes so the system kept working. There is strength in unity, and we understood that instinctively.

The walk home was much the same, though the cast of companions shifted. The children from my neighborhood mostly attended different schools, so my journey back was filled with classmates instead. At the end of the day, we would gather one another, knocking on classroom doors, collecting friends like beads on a string until the group was ready. And then we'd set out—singing, playing games, retelling the day's stories—before scattering again as each turned into their own neighborhood.

Afternoons belonged to us. After school, I spent hours with the neighborhood children—at the soccer field, in each other's courtyards, fishing at the nearby lake. Fishing was one of our few "nature" pastimes. Douala did not offer the kind of outdoor leisure I would later see abroad—no hiking trails, no managed mountain paths. The wilds of Cameroon were just that: wild, untamed, and often dangerous. So we found our wilderness in the middle of the city, on the banks of a lake where we cast our lines and felt, for a time, like adventurers.

Still, nothing compared to soccer. In Cameroon, soccer is more than a pastime—it is the heartbeat of the country. You begin as soon as you can walk, chasing a ball across dirt lots and concrete courtyards, and most never stop playing. Any open space could become a field. Pickup games formed at dusk, families gathering to cheer or join in.

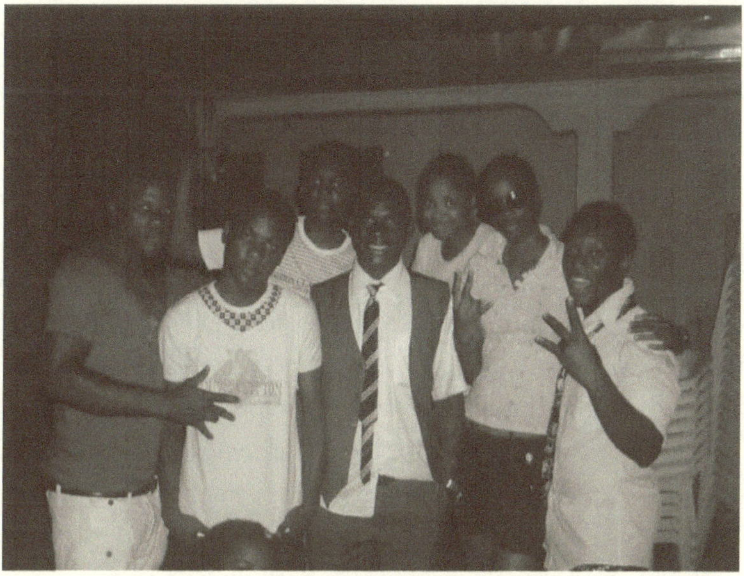

A bittersweet farewell captured in the heart of Kotto, Douala, Cameroon. Surrounded by the laughter and love of my childhood friends on one of my last days before embarking on a new life in the USA. This moment, at my younger brother's baptism, is a poignant reminder of my roots, the enduring power of friendship, and the courage it takes to chase your dreams across oceans.. From left to right; Charly (Gun), Joel (Baoba), Loic (Disco), Dimi (Sena), Nina, Edimo (Edims), Doudou (DDB).

Sometimes, we organized tournaments within our neighborhood. Older children played, younger ones watched. Everyone pitched in a small buy-in, and the winners split the pot. These were grand affairs in our eyes, but they seemed modest compared to the tournaments that pitted neighborhoods against one another. Every quarter of Douala had its own team, and once a year all twenty came together for the championship. Those matches were true events, drawing crowds from across the city. People traveled long distances to watch, to cheer, to bet. The buy-ins were larger, the prizes more significant, and for the players, it was a chance to be seen, to step onto a bigger stage.

Soccer was not just a game. It was how we measured ourselves, how we connected with our neighbors, how we tested our courage. It was the rhythm of our lives—woven into every childhood memory I carry from those long days in Douala.

It was a great honor to be chosen for your neighborhood team, but every child in Cameroon carried a dream far larger than the dusty fields where we played. We all looked to Europe, to the great leagues, and beyond them to the chance of wearing our nation's colors in the Olympics. It was the dream whispered on every pitch, the dream stitched into every goal scored at dusk. I, too, once carried it.

But for me, it faded sooner than it did for many of my friends. It wasn't that I stopped loving the game—I still loved it, still played in our neighborhood tournaments, still felt the rush when a ball rolled to my feet. It was simply that, as I grew older, other ambitions began to take hold. I was spared the ache that comes when childhood dreams collide with reality, when talent and opportunity prove unequal to desire. My heart began to turn elsewhere, toward something steadier: education.

In the beginning, school was just another excuse to be with my friends. The joy was in the company, in the long walks to and from the classrooms, in the chatter and the games we carried with us like contraband. But slowly, almost without me noticing, that shifted. My affection stretched beyond the friendships and into the subjects themselves.

In Cameroon, children begin elementary school at the age of two. My memories from those early years are scattered, more feeling than fact: crayons dulling against paper, shapes that refused to stay inside their outlines, colors shouted across the page, the sing-song repetition of words I was just learning to pronounce. Much of it was play, the kind of practice children everywhere know. By five, the lessons grew sharper—reading letters, tracing words, counting. By ten, we had glimpsed geography, touched lightly on the story of Cameroon itself, our history carried in short chapters and names we repeated until they settled in our mouths.

I began to notice, even then, that school came more easily to me than it did to many of my peers. Where they struggled, I understood; where they faltered, I remembered. Cameroon does not have the same structure of grade levels found in the West. Instead, you begin at a certain age and work steadily through subjects, passing national examinations as you are ready. My aptitude allowed me to advance quickly, and I left elementary school two years early to enter middle school. Still, at that stage, I was not working to my fullest. I did enough to keep my parents satisfied, enough to keep moving forward. The fire to learn for myself had not yet fully caught.

Middle school and high school were not separate institutions where I lived—they were housed in the same building, a single stretch of education that lasted roughly eight years. Most children began around thirteen. I started at nine. For me, the beginning of middle school was something like what Americans would call fifth grade. It was then that the difficulty sharpened, the work became real: mathematics that curled around itself into harder shapes, sciences that reached deeper, literature that pulled us into unfamiliar voices, history that demanded more than memorization. It was the start of the real journey, and I felt, for the first time, that learning itself could be a calling.

At the start of middle school, I didn't yet have a favorite subject. I enjoyed them all in their own way, though my father—who had studied marketing analysis in college—quietly pushed me toward mathematics. In Cameroon, parents make most of the decisions for their children, and my father's love of numbers was unshakable. If I ever mentioned something interesting I had learned in history or literature, he would smile, nod, and gently steer the conversation back to math and science.

I respected my parents deeply, and I think it was in those years that I first began to see numbers and formulas as the path to my future. I applied myself most in those subjects, and they came easily to me. So much so that in history class, while the teacher lectured, I would sometimes have my math notebook open, working through old problems or re-solving assignments just to test myself.

That was when my friends gave me my first nickname: Square Root. It was meant as a joke, but also as a compliment, and I wore it proudly. I was often the one tutoring them after school, helping with homework, or explaining lessons they hadn't grasped. I became, in their words, "like an assistant teacher." And because I never looked down on anyone for struggling, I grew into a kind of leadership role among my classmates—even though I was younger than all of them. That earned me another nickname: Sena, short for Senator.

But as much as I thrived, I knew the system around me was broken. I've already spoken of medicine as one of Cameroon's great challenges. The other is education.

Primary schooling falls into three categories: public, private, or none at all. And "none" was heartbreakingly common. About half the children in my neighborhood—some of my closest friends—couldn't go to school. Even public schools required a fee, roughly twenty U.S. dollars per semester, and for many families, that was impossible. But instead of creating social divides, the absence of schooling shaped a different response. In Cameroon, there was no bitterness, no contempt. If one family managed to send a child to school, it was celebrated, not envied. It was seen as a victory for the whole neighborhood, an improvement for the family we all belonged to.

Still, even those who could pay were not guaranteed a quality education. My siblings and I all attended public school, and we only succeeded because my parents filled the gaps. Classrooms often held over a hundred students for a single teacher. Those teachers were underpaid, overworked, and starved of resources. There were no computers in the classrooms, no chemistry labs stocked with beakers and burners, no televisions with lessons queued up. Learning was chalk on a board, paper on a desk, and a teacher doing their best against impossible odds.

That was where my parents stepped in. After working long hours—sometimes until nine at night—they still found time to sit with us, to go over lessons, to demand more from us than our schools could. My mother, especially, poured herself into that work. She had always dreamed of being a teacher, and in us, she found her students. Helping with our homework lit something in her; it was her joy as much as her duty.

Her greatest invention was her reward system. She wanted us to see that effort led to results, and results brought rewards. So whenever we performed well on an exam, she gave us a small monetary prize. For me, already a little miser in training, it was all the motivation I needed. I would save every franc, slipping it into the wooden safe under my bed. And so I studied hard, not only for knowledge, not only for my parents' approval, but also for the quiet pleasure of hearing the coins clink into my box. By the end of each term, I was wealthier in knowledge and in savings. By the end of each year, I had proof that effort bore fruit.

And in this way, I grew—into the boy called Square Root, into the Senator of my peers, and into the student my parents hoped I would become.

Even with my parents' dedication, they knew the limits of what public schooling in Cameroon could provide. They could see that their children—especially me—would never fully reach their potential in classrooms so crowded, with resources so thin. I was the quickest to grasp lessons, the most eager of my siblings, and I think my parents felt the weight of that truth most heavily with me. That is why, before my second year of middle school, they made the decision to transfer me into private school.

It was no small feat. They had saved diligently through the success of their businesses, sacrificing comforts in order to give us something more. And for me, the difference was felt immediately.

In public school, the challenge was simply survival—trying to hear the teacher's words in a classroom of one hundred voices, trying to learn without books or equipment. In private school, the challenge was different. There were more teachers, smaller classes, and better resources. For the first time, I found myself pressed by the work itself. For the first time, I had to struggle.

I won't say I loved it at once. The assignments consumed more of my day and pulled me away from time with my friends. But even then, I could sense the benefit. I could see how this sharpened me, and how it allowed me to return the favor to my siblings and friends, helping them in their own studies. Soon enough, the rigor became something I enjoyed for its own sake.

It was also around this time that faith began to take deeper root in me. My family was strict in our attendance—we went to church every Sunday, and my father served as an elder in our Evangelical Protestant congregation. I remember one sermon in particular. The pastor spoke about how Christians were not meant merely to survive, not to shuffle through life placing one foot ahead of the other, but to strive for excellence, to be "the head and not the tail." Those words landed heavily. At a time when I was just beginning to delight in my studies, they gave me purpose. If learning was my path, then I was called to walk it with excellence.

By the time I reached the equivalent of eighth grade, another choice presented itself. In Cameroon, every student must choose a foreign language. And in ninth, a specialty—a track that shapes your education into literature, accounting, science, and so forth. My father, true to form, chose for me. He selected science, the path with the most math and the least of everything else. But by then, it was no longer just his will guiding me. What had begun as a desire to please my parents had grown into a true passion.

I devoured my math and science notebooks, covering pages with equations and diagrams until my mother sometimes had to intervene. When I neglected my chores or failed to give attention to other subjects, she punished me not by adding labor, but by taking those notebooks away. That was the greatest punishment she could imagine for me, and the greatest I could feel.

In those years, I began to understand not only the direction of my education but the joy of discipline, the way passion can be shaped into purpose.

I was the first experiment in private school, and the experiment worked. Two years after my transfer, my parents enrolled the rest of my siblings, and each of us benefited from the stricter structure and better resources that environment provided.

But a distinction must be made. Even private school in Cameroon bore little resemblance to public schools in places like the United States. There was no air conditioning to blunt the thick heat. There were no desks arranged neatly in rows. Instead, students sat shoulder to shoulder on wooden benches, balancing notebooks on our laps while the teacher wrote on the chalkboard. There were no individual textbooks. Each of us carried a notebook for every subject, and when the teacher spoke, we scribbled as fast as our hands could move. Those pages were our lifeline; our notes became the only material we had to study from later.

There were no janitors either. On Fridays, students cleaned the classrooms ourselves—sweeping the floors, wiping down the teacher's desk, polishing the windows. And there were no extracurricular activities to balance the long academic days. No clubs, no teams, no student governments or debate societies. School was school, nothing more. Classes began at seven in the morning and ended at five in the evening, broken only by a half-hour for lunch. Then we went home. That was the rhythm of our lives.

Private schools, to their credit, were slightly more organized than the public system. Once or twice a year, they might host events for the students. One such occasion was National Youth Week in February, when our school held a festival of music and celebration. But those were exceptions. For the most part, our days were strict and studious, year after year.

The academic calendar ran from September through May, divided into three trimesters. National exams marked the transitions. There were four in all, given at points roughly equivalent to moving from third to fourth grade, sixth to seventh, eleventh to twelfth, and finally from secondary school into university. But they were not tied to age. Parents registered their children when they believed they were ready. If you failed, you repeated the subjects and tried again. Many students were held back this way, and many never made it beyond primary school—especially those in public education.

Even with such high attrition, the universities overflowed. There were only a handful in Cameroon, and gaining entry was fiercely competitive. After passing the national exam, you still had to sit for each university's own entrance test, no matter what degree you hoped to pursue. The burden was so heavy that most students applied to only one or two schools at most.

But I never had to face that struggle. My parents had a different vision. Their ambition was not simply that we survive the Cameroonian system, but that we rise beyond it. From an early age, they promised us that if we excelled in our studies, they would help us pursue higher education in the United States. That promise became my compass. It was the image I held before me through every long day of class, every late-night study session, every examination. It was the lighthouse that guided me through the storms of my schooling, urging me always to push harder, to aim higher.

And with that promise in hand, I did exactly that.

3

CULTURE SHOCK

MOST PEOPLE DO NOT REALIZE how difficult it is for someone outside the United States to enter, even when the goal is only to study and not to naturalize. I was sixteen when I graduated high school in Cameroon and began that process with my parents. I cannot recall every detail now, but what lingers in memory is the weight of it—the way it felt less like applying for school and more like being vetted by an intelligence agency.

The documentation seemed endless. There were the obvious requirements: a birth certificate, proof of vaccinations, proof of graduation. But there were so many others I had never imagined. I had to provide transcripts from every year of schooling, reaching all the way back to elementary. Letters were needed from teachers. My parents had to turn over their financial records. I was even subjected to a medical examination and rounds of bloodwork. The message was clear: the United States was not interested in simply letting anyone in. They wanted healthy, motivated individuals who would contribute immediately.

It took us a month just to prepare the paperwork. Then we drove six hours to Yaoundé, the capital, to file at the U.S. Embassy. After submitting everything, I waited only one day for the answer: I had been accepted. I remember the joy of that moment, the way it filled me with certainty that the hardest part was over. But I was wrong. The visa was only the beginning. I still needed a passport. From start to finish, the process of leaving Cameroon and stepping onto a plane stretched nearly five months—and that was considered the expedited path.

The flight itself was unlike anything I had ever known. It was my first time on an airplane, and the experience was overwhelming. The hum of engines, the flashing of warning lights, the strict instructions delivered in clipped tones—all of it pressed against my nerves. I had heard the horror stories of planes going down over the ocean, and so I prayed constantly. A prayer for takeoff. A prayer for landing. Another for every stretch of the long, twenty-four-hour journey.

And then there was the sound of the cabin: a chorus of languages swirling around me—French, English, Spanish, German, Chinese, and others I did not recognize. Everyone else seemed so at ease, slipping into their seats as though they had always belonged there. I, meanwhile, sat stiff, wide-eyed, feeling like the only stranger in a world where everyone else knew the rules.

At sixteen, it was the first time in my life I can remember feeling truly isolated—truly alone.

My first flight was not all nerves and fear. It was, in truth, a balance—a mixture of emotions both welcome and unwelcome, hope braided with anxiety. At the airport, my family gathered to send me off. It was a ritual already established with my older brothers when they left for the United States. My mother and father, my younger brother and sister, aunts and uncles, cousins, grandparents—everyone was there. Their faces shone with pride, but their eyes glistened with tears. We embraced, exchanged kisses, and then I walked alone toward the security check. I was younger than my brothers had been when they left, and I could feel in the heaviness of those goodbyes how difficult it was for them to watch me go.

But I had prepared myself. I carried pictures—of family, of friends, of the places I knew by heart—knowing I would need them when the ache of distance came. I packed carefully, aware that I was leaving behind everything familiar with no certain idea of when I might return. Snacks filled my bag, to be eaten before landing since customs would not allow them through. Clothes and supplies were folded in, enough to last for months, because my brothers had warned me of the cost of life in America. Even with their advice, the reality would still startle me.

Once I settled into my seat and my nerves eased, I began to enjoy the wonder of the journey. I had a window seat, and I spent hours staring out at the world below. The view was more breathtaking than I had ever imagined—the vast, endless sweep of sky, the oceans and landmasses stretched beneath the wing. I could not look away. My route on Ethiopian Airlines took me from Douala to Addis Ababa, then to Rome, and finally across the Atlantic to Washington,

D.C. Each leg of the journey felt like stepping further into another life.

When the Atlantic ended and the American skyline rose out of the horizon, my heart beat with equal parts excitement and fear. My brothers were already there—Landry, who had been in the U.S. for three years, and Wilfried, for one. I had not seen either of them since they left, and the thought of being reunited filled me with joy. At the same time, I was restless, anxious to discover what my life would look like in this new place.

But the moment my feet touched the ground at Dulles International Airport, I realized how greatly I had underestimated the difference between my home and here. In an instant, I felt the immensity of the distance—not only in miles, but in culture, language, and atmosphere. It was the beginning of a new life, and though I did not yet understand it, that life would shape me in ways I could never have imagined.

I remember stepping off the plane, at first overwhelmed with excitement by the scene unfolding around me. The terminal seemed alive, like a great street festival—people streaming through corridors from every direction, voices echoing, bags rolling. What a welcome, I thought. But soon the energy shifted. I began to see that for all their numbers, none of these people truly saw each other. They moved quickly, eyes fixed forward, shoulders brushing without acknowledgment. Even in the gate I had just left behind, where travelers sat in rows of chairs waiting for their own departures, not a single glance rose from a book or fell from the televisions hanging overhead.

Children squirmed in their seats, restless. When one dared to break free, a parent would snatch them back, pressing them into place and then apologizing to those nearby, as if their child had committed a theft. It was a choreography of order and silence I had never witnessed before.

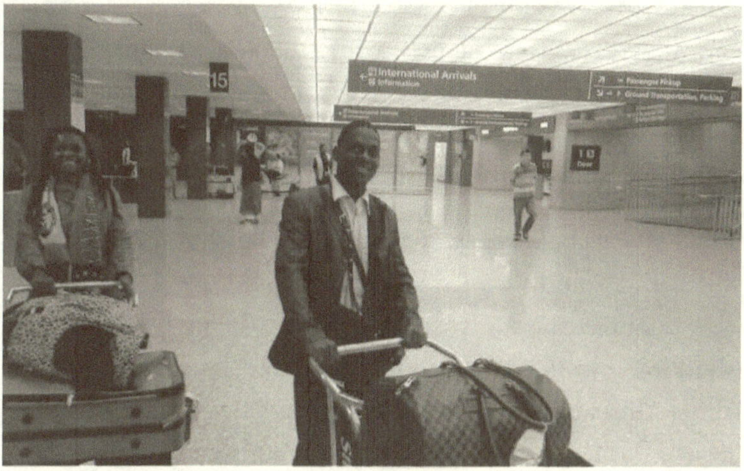

A single step, a giant leap towards a new destiny. Arriving at Dulles International Airport in Virginia, my first day in the USA. This image marks the beginning of a transformative journey, filled with hope, uncertainty, and the promise of new opportunities. It represents the courage to leave the familiar behind and embrace the challenges and rewards of starting anew in a foreign land.

I stepped into the main corridor smiling, my instinctive greeting to any who might meet my eye. But those who did either looked away quickly, pretending not to see, or gave me a puzzled glance, as if wondering what I wanted from them. That was the first moment I realized how deeply our gestures of warmth, the habits I carried without thought, marked me as different here. In Cameroon, you greet everyone—friend, neighbor, stranger. In America, I found myself choking back a thousand hellos, holding my arms tight to my sides to keep them from waving, swallowing the impulse to embrace a stranger or kiss their cheek.

If the behavior of the people was startling, the airport itself was astonishing. Everywhere I turned, digital screens flashed with flight statuses. Endless lines of passengers wound toward counters to check bags or claim tickets. Terminals multiplied, gates stretched without end, and mechanized walkways carried people swiftly from one place to another. I felt as though I had not simply crossed into another country but into another century, into the future.

I had always believed Douala was a great city, sprawling and alive. But standing in that airport, the place I had always called home suddenly felt small, fragile in comparison. I shuddered to think of Landry, my eldest brother, navigating all of this alone when he first arrived years earlier. The thought of being the only soul you knew in a place so vast—I wasn't sure I could have borne it.

Fortunately, I would not have to.

Through the labyrinth of corridors, I collected my bags and stepped out into the arrival area. And there was Landry. Relief washed over me at the sight of his familiar face. We embraced, and soon we were driving away, heading toward Gaithersburg, Maryland, to the apartment he shared with Wilfried and our cousin. That small apartment became my home—for six years, the first chapter of my American life.

I had always gotten along with my siblings. Being the middle of five gave me a unique perspective—I was the youngest of the oldest and the oldest of the youngest, a bridge between two halves of the family. I could understand both sides, and often found myself playing the role of mediator. But moving in with my older brothers in America, without the steady hand of our parents, introduced new challenges.

In Cameroon, the oldest sibling takes on the role of parent whenever the real parents are absent. It is not mere bossiness; it is part of the culture, reinforced by elders and expected of everyone. When we were young, if our parents were late coming home from work, Landry bore the responsibility for keeping order—making sure we shared, helped each other, and followed the rules of the house. And we respected him in that role. I looked up to Landry, and when our parents moved an ocean away, that dynamic only deepened. In America, he became, in many ways, my new father. And he took that responsibility seriously.

He had reason to. By the time I arrived, Landry had already been in the United States for years. He and Wilfried had jobs, paid their bills, managed their lives. They were, for all intents and purposes, adults. I, on the other hand, was sixteen—fresh from Cameroon, without a job, without bearings, wide-eyed and disoriented in this new culture. Landry, naturally, saw me as a child. The problem was, I no longer saw myself that way. I had finished high school, was on the threshold of college, and believed I had earned the right to independence in my decisions. That difference in perception created friction between us, and as I grew older and more self-reliant, the friction only increased.

Some conflicts were ordinary, the kind you might expect when young men share a space together. We had to learn respect for each other's belongings—especially food. We had to figure out how to keep the apartment clean, how to split bills fairly, how to live as a unit without driving each other mad.

But for me, the greatest pressure point was financial. Almost immediately, I realized I needed a job. Part of it was practical: America was expensive, far more than I had ever imagined. Part of it was personal: I wanted to contribute, to pull my own weight, to be treated not as a child but as an equal. And part of it was survival: if I wanted to preserve the closeness I had always shared with my brothers, I needed time away from the apartment. Too much proximity risked wearing down the bond that had carried us across an ocean.

Work, then, was not just about money. It was about respect, about independence, about becoming who I needed to be in this new world.

Coming from not only a completely different culture but also from a life where nearly all of my needs were still provided by my parents, I was stunned at the cost of even the most basic things in America. In Douala, the best quality gallon of milk cost around 500 CFA—barely one U.S. dollar. In the United States, the cheapest gallon was twice that, not even including tax. Toothpaste back home was the equivalent of twenty cents; a good pair of shoes could be had for four dollars. Our thrift shops sold used and surplus American clothes, and for a dollar apiece you could walk away with pants, shirts, jackets—enough to fill a wardrobe. College books in Cameroon, even the most expensive, rarely cost more than twenty dollars. In America, the cheapest used book I could find was a hundred. But the most astonishing of all were haircuts and grooming products. In Cameroon, the very best haircut cost no more than thirty cents, a bottle of shampoo fifty, a razor ten. In America, those same things seemed to belong to another world entirely.

When I began working, I couldn't stop making comparisons in my head—measuring what I could have bought in Cameroon for the same wages I was earning here. It became a quiet burden, both mental and emotional. How, I wondered, could anyone make a living in this country? How would I ever earn enough to stand on my own?

My first job was cleaning offices, working for a company owned by fellow African expatriates. I was sixteen, still unable to speak English, and it was the only work I could find. I was not particularly skilled at cleaning, but I was grateful. Most of my coworkers were also Africans, many of them students, and in those early months their presence offered me a kind of comfort—familiar voices and familiar manners in a place that felt so foreign. The pay was low, about two hundred dollars a month, but I handed all of it to Landry to help with the bills. Even then, it was never enough. There were times when we fell behind, and those late notices in the mail were another kind of culture shock.

In Cameroon, if you needed something, you asked. Everyone knew one another's struggles and dreams, and those struggles and dreams belonged to the entire community. If a family was short on food, a neighbor provided. If a tool was needed, another lent it. We belonged to each other. But here, in America, it seemed as though everyone lived behind invisible walls. You might not even know the name of the person living across the hall. Asking a neighbor for sugar, let alone for money, felt unthinkable. My neighborhood, once a network of thousands, had shrunk to four people in one apartment. The loneliness of that realization pressed heavily on me.

And with that loneliness came pressure. Landry, stepping into the role of father, expected me to bring in more money. I was already attending an English Language Institute by day and cleaning at night, but I understood his demands. Hard work was the rhythm of life in Cameroon. Unemployment was not a concept we grew up with—if you could work, you worked. You did whatever was available for whatever it paid until something better appeared. And so I resolved to do the same here. I would work more, I would study harder, and I would find my footing. Because I needed not only to survive, but to belong.

After I graduated from the English Language Institute, I enrolled in basic classes at the Community College in Rockville, Maryland. I was eager to begin—education was the very reason I had come to America—but what I hadn't realized was that stepping into college would also unlock new opportunities for work. To my surprise, I found it remarkably easy to secure jobs on campus. I was hired in the library and also as a math tutor. It was ideal: no long commutes, no juggling schedules between school and employment. I could simply walk from class to work along the same sidewalks.

The pay was better, too. Between the two jobs I worked close to thirty hours a week, and my earnings jumped from two hundred dollars a month to six hundred. That increase felt like sunlight breaking through after a long storm. For the first time, the bills were fully covered, and I felt like an equal contributor in the household. Life became lighter for all of us. Still, even with triple the income of my first job, there was nothing left to save. Every dollar went to living expenses, and the inability to put anything aside gnawed at me. I was used to saving, even as a child, and I longed to build a small reserve. So I kept searching for more.

First, I started tutoring privately. Instead of going through the college, I charged students directly, cutting out the middle institution. My hourly rate rose sharply, and that helped. Then I applied for work as a therapist for autistic children—teaching basic math, social skills, and behavioral practices. To my surprise, I excelled at it. I connected deeply with the families and felt, maybe for the first time, that my work had a real and immediate impact. It awakened in me a passion I hadn't anticipated, a sense that helping others could be just as fulfilling as solving equations on paper.

With these changes, I finally began to breathe. I could pay my share of the rent and bills, buy small things for myself, and even tuck money away for future needs. The relief was immense. But it was short-lived.

Community college was supposed to be a two-year program, but I had already fallen behind. Adjusting to a new language and culture while working so many hours meant I took fewer classes than I should have. That alone weighed on me—I felt like I wasn't meeting my own expectations. Then came the news that shook me. My parents, back in Cameroon, could no longer cover my tuition. Their businesses had slowed, their earnings dropped, and with several siblings also in school, there was no longer enough to go around. Worse still, I already owed money from previous semesters. Until those debts were cleared, I could not re-enroll.

It hit me like a blow. My dream had been so clear: to come to America, to study, to earn the education that would open every door. I had already come so far—left my family, crossed an ocean, learned a new language, taken my first steps in college. And now, suddenly, the path was blocked. I remember feeling adrift, uncertain, and profoundly lost.

Around that time, tensions in the apartment began to rise. My older brother grew more insistent, more controlling—or at least that was how it felt to me then. Looking back, perhaps he hadn't changed at all. Perhaps it was I who had changed, growing more independent, less tolerant of being told what to do. He would dictate when I needed to be home and, if I argued, remind me that I was to respect him because he was in charge, responsible for my safety. But by then, those words rang hollow. I no longer believed I needed protection. I was sixteen, handling my own finances, making my own decisions. I was not a child in need of another parent.

With school temporarily out of reach, I found myself with both time on my hands and a strong desire to spend less of it inside that apartment. I began searching for something meaningful to do, some way to regain the sense of belonging I had always known in Cameroon's extended family life. That is how I came to apply as a volunteer at Asbury Methodist Village, a local nursing home. To my relief, they welcomed me in.

I became a resident's assistant, and my work was simple: fetching water, delivering newspapers, running small errands, escorting patients where they needed to go. Yet the heart of the job was not in the tasks—it was in the time spent sitting with residents, listening to their stories, offering company. That was what they needed most, and it was what I most enjoyed giving. Slowly, I built lasting friendships within those walls, and in helping others, I felt my own footing return.

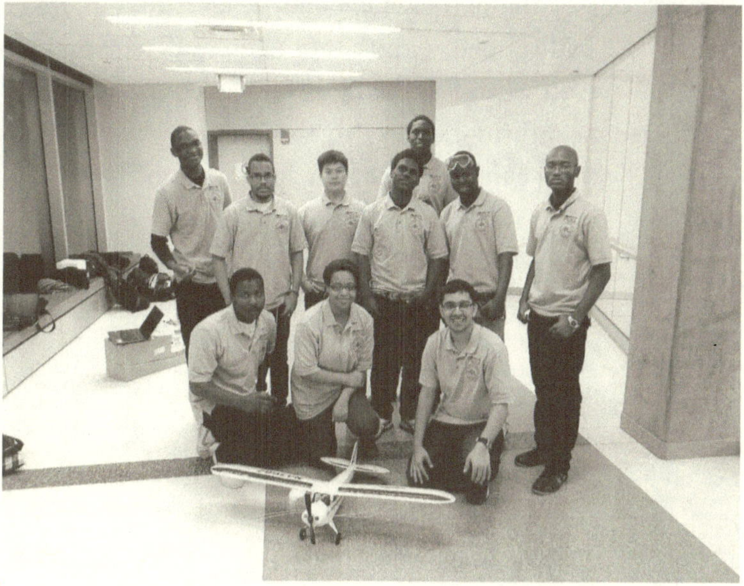

Igniting innovation: As part of Montgomery College's MESA (Math, Engineering, and Science Achievement) program, underrepresented engineering students, including myself, designed and built groundbreaking solutions to real-world societal challenges. Our projects were a testament to the power of diverse minds solving critical problems and a step on our own paths to purpose.

The work gave me clarity. With a little money saved, I went back to the community college to speak with a counselor, prepared for disappointment. Instead, I was surprised to learn there was a way forward: a new payment plan with smaller installments spread over time. Within a single semester, I was back in school. Scholarships followed, helping to ease some of what I already owed. In time, I earned my two-year degree and was accepted into the University of Maryland at College Park to study Biomedical Engineering.

But Asbury never left me. Volunteering there had carried me through one of the hardest moments of my young life, and the bond I had formed with the residents was too strong to let go. So even as my academic workload grew heavier, I continued to return—because in those quiet conversations and small acts of care, I felt part of a family again.

4

PURPOSE

THE UNIVERSITY OF MARYLAND at College Park was an easy choice. It was close enough to Gaithersburg that I could continue living with my brothers and cousin, postponing the need to strike out entirely on my own. By then, I had saved enough from my jobs to buy a car, and the short commute posed no difficulty.

Choosing a major, however, was not so simple. I loved math and felt at home in the sciences, but that still left a wide horizon of possibilities. My parents had always urged me toward either engineering or medicine, and I had considered both in broad terms, though I had never been sure which direction pulled me most.

At the same time, my experiences outside of the classroom had left their mark. Working as an autism therapist, and even more profoundly, volunteering at Asbury, had awakened something new in me—a growing desire to work with people, to play some role in their healing and in the improvement of their lives. I wanted my future to blend knowledge with compassion, precision with purpose.

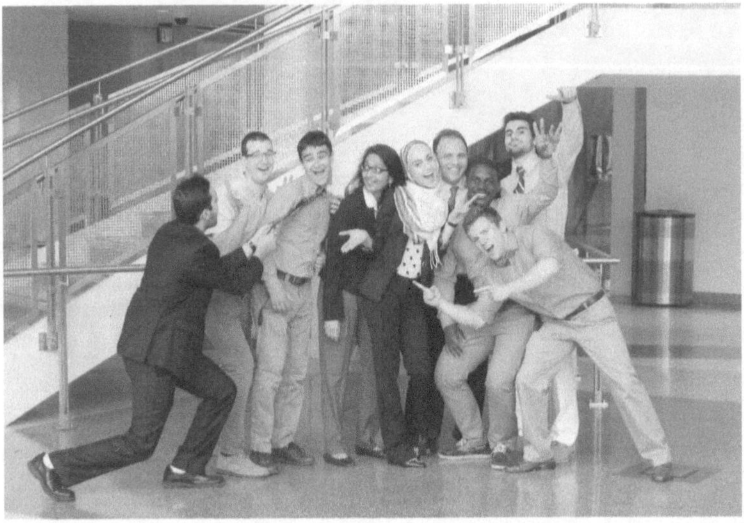

Graduation from the University of Maryland College Park, a milestone shared with some of my biomedical engineering friends.

It was during this search that I first discovered Biomedical Engineering. I had never heard of it before, but the name alone seemed to bridge my two worlds: engineering and medicine. The program promised a heavy focus on math and science—subjects I loved—and minimal emphasis on literature courses, which suited me well. More than that, I learned that many students in the program went on to pursue medicine after their degree. That possibility, of keeping both paths open until I was ready to choose, appealed to me deeply.

So I applied, and I was accepted. Once again, scholarships helped ease the way, but tuition was far more expensive than community college had been. Reducing my work schedule was not an option. If anything, I had to maintain my hours even as the workload increased.

Still, when classes began, I found my rhythm. I loved the coursework, and for the first time since arriving in America, I began to build friendships with people my own age outside of work and volunteering. We studied together, shared the same pressures, compared notes on the same challenges. I joined study groups, laughed between lectures, and even began to spend time with classmates beyond the campus walls.

For years, my life had been divided between survival and obligation—family, work, bills. At College Park, I began to glimpse something different: a sense of belonging, not just in America, but among peers who were walking the same road I was.

Even as my studies at Maryland grew more demanding, I continued to volunteer at Asbury Methodist Village. By then, it had become less of a volunteer post and more of a second home, a place where I felt anchored. It also gave me a small but meaningful glimpse into medical care in the United States. Though it was a nursing home, doctors came regularly to check on residents, to diagnose persistent conditions, to prescribe new treatments. I would watch closely as they made their rounds, listening to how they spoke with patients, how they carried themselves. I learned more in those quiet moments of observation than I could have from any textbook.

It was after one such visit that I noticed a woman I had grown close to behaving differently. She was Asian, probably in her sixties, and over the years I had formed a warm bond with her. But on that day, she was unlike herself. Her eyes were fixed on the floor, her movements slow. Normally she would greet me with a smile, or at least with words, but now she sat silent, staring at the wall as though I wasn't even there.

I asked gently if she was alright, if there was something I could do. Nothing. I stepped closer, placed a hand on her shoulder, and asked again. This time she lifted her gaze, and I could see the fear swimming in her eyes. A doctor had told her earlier that she would need surgery the next morning—an amputation. Diabetes had already caused her many complications, but this was the most serious yet. Her voice trembled as she explained, and I realized she had no one—no family to sit with her that night, no visitor to hold her hand before or after, no one to wait for her in the hospital.

I stayed with her for hours. At first, she spoke haltingly, circling back to the surgery, her illness, her fear. But as time passed, her words softened. She began sharing stories from her life, small memories, fragments of her childhood. By the end of the evening she was smiling, even laughing, teasing me about my accent, listening as I told her stories of my own—about the mischief of my siblings, about soccer games in Cameroon. It was as much therapy for me as it was for her. We were two people far from our families, finding comfort in each other's presence.

Before I left that night, I told her I would be with her the next day, at the hospital, for the surgery. I had never done anything like that for a resident before. I don't know exactly what moved me to it—perhaps I imagined myself in her place, or perhaps I thought of my mother one day facing such a moment alone. Whatever the reason, I knew it was the right thing.

The following morning, the surgery went ahead without complications. I was there as I had promised. She remained calm throughout, her spirits lifted, her smile never far from her lips—even as she came to terms with the loss of her limb.

During my final years at Asbury, I grew closer to many of the residents, but eventually the demands of school and work overtook me, and I had to stop volunteering. On my last day, one of the women I had bonded with most deeply stopped me before I left. She told me something I have never forgotten.

She said that in all her years at Asbury, with doctors and nurses and volunteers passing through, I was the only one who had ever treated her as a person first and a patient second.

At the time, I brushed it off as kindness. I thanked her, smiled, and carried the words lightly. But over time, her compliment began to grow inside me like a seed. Slowly, it took root. Slowly, it began to shape me. By the time I reached the end of my bachelor's program, it had become one of the strongest motivators in my life.

I realized that what she had said was more than a compliment—it was a calling. She had not said simply "person," but "patient" as well. She had seen me not only as a caring presence, but as a professional. That dual recognition meant everything. It drew me back to my memories of the Mercy Ships in Cameroon—the doctors who treated me, who treated countless others with dignity, bringing healing and joy into places where there had been only fear. I wanted to be that. I wanted to help people in that same way.

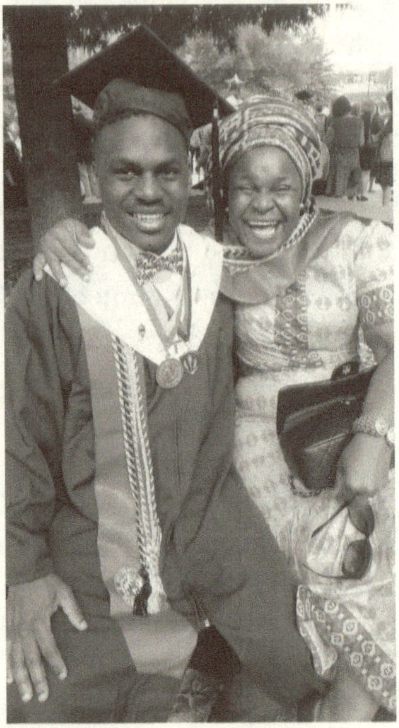

Behind every dream fulfilled, there is unwavering support and boundless love. Standing beside my mother at my graduation ceremony from the University of Maryland College Park, I felt the weight of years of shared sacrifice, encouragement, and belief. This moment wasn't just my achievement; it was our achievement, a powerful testament to the impact of familial love in shaping a journey to purpose.

And so, in my final year at Maryland, I leaned toward medicine. A friend in my program introduced me to his father, a practicing doctor, and when I asked if I might shadow him, he welcomed me. That semester, I spent as much time in his office as I could. I greeted patients, took their histories, listened as they explained their symptoms. I observed the doctor's methods—how he decided on treatment plans, how he balanced science with empathy. And I discovered, to my surprise and delight, that I was completely at ease in that environment. I loved it. I was comfortable with patients, confident in the work, and inspired by the responsibility of medicine. That was when I knew with certainty: my future lay not in engineering, but in medicine.

When my shadowing ended, my friend's father wrote me a recommendation letter for medical school, and I felt ready to begin the next chapter. But almost immediately, I stumbled.

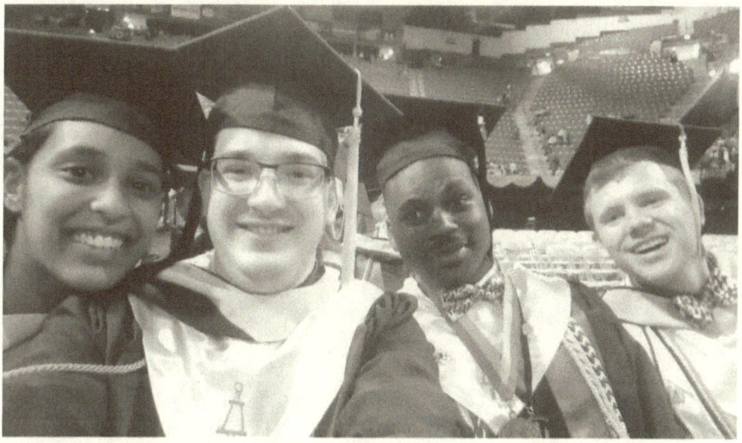

Celebrating the culmination of hard work and shared dreams. Biomedical Engineering Graduation day at the University of Maryland, College Park. A selfie with my friends, the brilliant minds with whom I navigated the challenges of academia and the excitement of scientific discovery. This image captures the joy of achievement, the bonds of camaraderie, and the hopeful anticipation of applying our knowledge to make a difference in the world. From left to right, Lily Peterken, Bryan Pinsky, myself, Kevin Pineault.

I can't recall exactly what I had expected from the medical school application process—only that whatever I thought it would be, the reality was much harder. Community college had been simple: proof of high school graduation, a visa, a check, and I was enrolled. Even my transfer to Maryland had not been especially difficult. The hardest part had been securing scholarships, but the admissions process itself was straightforward.

Medical school, however, was something else entirely.

Applying to medical school was an entirely different animal. It felt, in many ways, like going through the process of coming to the United States all over again—only this time, I didn't even know where to begin.

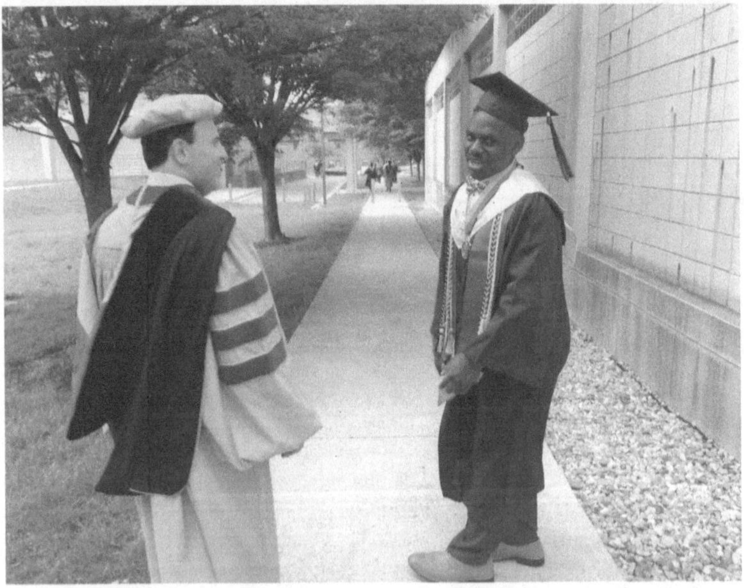

Captured by my mother on the walk to my graduation ceremony, this moment with my UMD mentor, Peter Kofinas, PhD, who guided me through medical school applications, marks a significant step in my journey to purpose.

I started by asking my friends from Biomedical Engineering, most of whom were American-born. I was struck by how effortlessly they spoke about the process, as if they had been born knowing it. In truth, much of that knowledge had been absorbed by osmosis—through families with doctors, through years of growing up in this system, through conversations at dinner tables and casual advice from relatives. I, on the other hand, was starting from nothing. There were no doctors in my family. Not even healers. I had to build my understanding from the ground up.

I asked questions, met with admissions counselors, and tried to assemble the puzzle. But every conversation seemed to end with another list of things I hadn't yet done. *"Have you completed this step?"* No. *"Well then you can't move on to that step until you've done this one first. Better get started, because once that's done, you'll need to do the next."* The process spiraled endlessly, and my head spun trying to keep track of it all.

Eventually, I learned that all of these steps, all of these forms and prerequisites, funneled toward one thing: the Medical College Admission Test—the MCAT.

Years have passed since then, and time has dulled the sting enough that I can say it plainly now: the MCAT is a very hard test. The short version is this—I registered, studied, prepared, and took it. And I failed. Not in the sense of leaving it blank or walking out, but in the sense that my score was so low that not a single medical school in the country would consider me.

The truth is, I knew the material. I was strong in math and science. But English was still a second language, and the speed required to process the questions, understand their nuance, and answer within the strict time limits was too much.

That was one of the hardest moments of my life. I was in the final year of my Biomedical Engineering program, fully invested in the dream of pursuing medicine. My family had poured money, hope, and sacrifice into this dream. I had given seven years of my life to reach this point. And now, with one score sheet, it all seemed to collapse.

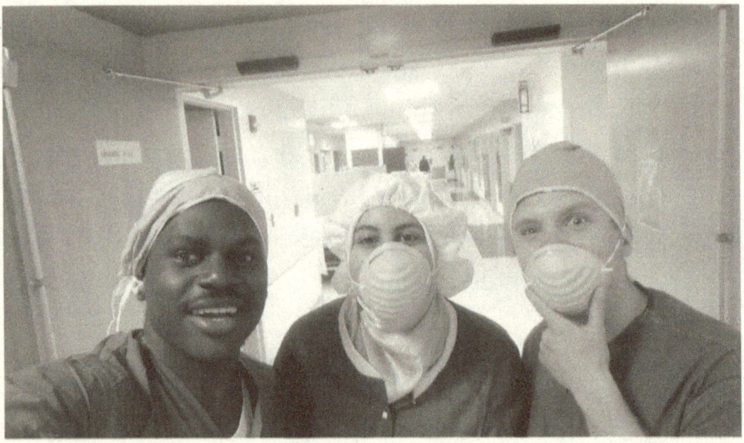

The first glimpse into the intricate dance of surgery. As a 4th year undergraduate student, standing with friends after observing my first surgical case at the University of Maryland Medical Center. From left to right, myself, Nadia Abutaleb, Kevin Pineault.

I leaned on those around me—my family, my friends, doctors I had come to know. They told me what I did not yet know myself: that many students fail the MCAT the first time, and that it was not the end. Their encouragement kept me from giving up. I resolved to try again.

This time I studied harder than I had ever studied for anything in my life. I also spent countless hours sharpening my English, drilling passages, practicing under time limits, teaching myself how to think in a new rhythm. When I sat for the exam a second time, I felt more confident. I understood the pacing, the topics, the pressure. I walked out of the testing center believing I had done well.

And I had. My score rose significantly. But it was still not enough. Not enough to open the doors I needed.

I remember staring at that results sheet for nearly an hour, numb. I was a good student. I was intelligent, hardworking, and excelling in my classes. I had pursued medicine for the right reasons—for people, for service, for care. And still, it was not enough to carry me across the line.

Believing I had run out of options, I decided that I would finish out my degree program and that would be it. I would pursue a career in the field of Biomedical Engineering. I took some time to get my mind right, focused on my classes and started talking to people about possible careers in Biomed. And that's when something amazing happened.

I was speaking to a friend in the program that I had thought was not planning to pursue medicine after graduation, but to my surprise he told me that he was, in fact, going on to study medicine—osteopathic medicine.

I'm ashamed to admit that until that moment, I could not remember ever having heard the words osteopathic medicine uttered before in my life. Somehow, in all my research about future career options in medicine, I had skipped over it entirely. It had never even come up during my time shadowing. How could that be? Before my friend had even finished telling me about it, I was already hooked.

He told me osteopathic medicine was a holistic approach to medicine, that its practitioners address all the systems of the body. They have the same knowledge that traditional medical doctors have. In fact, they are medical doctors, but they don't just stop at symptoms, illnesses, and prescriptions; they look at lifestyle, family dynamics, finances, exercise, stress, diet, and yes, diagnosable aspects of the person's immediate health. In short, they treat everyone individually, as a patient and as a person. I couldn't believe I hadn't heard of it before, and more, I couldn't believe how perfect it was for me and everything I wanted to do in medicine. This was what brought me to medicine in the first place, the desire to treat people as their whole selves, not just as numbers on a chart, or as diseases to solve. I wanted to help people become whole again.

The more my friend told me about the philosophy of osteopathic medicine, the more I fell in love with it; the idea that you could help the patient with not just medications, but also with your hands, your voice, your compassion, just being there for them—it was perfect.

But then my stomach sank as I remembered, I had already taken the MCAT twice. I'd given it my best shot and hadn't earned a single acceptance letter from a single medical school.

That's when my friend told me one of the most amazing things I had yet heard. Osteopathic medicine programs approach their applicants the same way their doctors approach their patients—individually, holistically. They don't just look at the MCAT. They also look at GPA. They also interview the applicant and get to know them. They want to know why they even want to pursue medicine in the first place. They look at the story of the applicant. They look at every case as an applicant and as a person, and that becomes the basis for their decision.

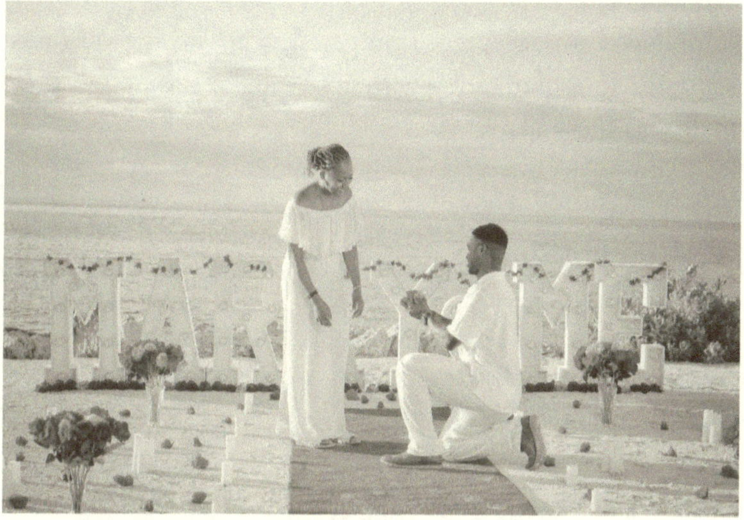

Against the backdrop of the breathtaking beauty of Montego Bay, Jamaica, I asked the most important question of my life. The day I proposed to my future wife, Anita. This image encapsulates a moment of pure joy, love, and the promise of a shared future. It's a reminder that amidst the demands of a physician's journey, there is always room for profound personal happiness and connection.

So, with renewed hope, I researched and applied to several schools of Osteopathic Medicine, and to my great surprise and delight, I received multiple invitations to interview. That alone, was further than I had gotten with schools of traditional medicine.

During the interview process, I received multiple offers, and ultimately decided to attend the West Virginia School of Osteopathic Medicine. It was close to where I lived, so again, I didn't have to move. But, more than anything else, I felt at home from my very first visit there. The woman who conducted the admissions interview made me feel like I was in the exact place I needed to be.

I applied. I got accepted. I prepared to attend the very next semester after graduating with my bachelor's. Now, all I had to do was succeed.

5

POSTERCHILD

Coming into my first year of medical school, and having performed so poorly in the MCAT, I was terrified that I would not succeed. I had never suffered an academic letdown like that, and I think it shook my confidence quite a bit. This was not helped by the amount of pressure placed on me by my parents, siblings, and other loved ones back in Cameroon. In Cameroon culture, everyone expects a great deal of those who are able to study in other countries, the U.S. especially. Back home, your parents give updates to others in the neighborhood where you grew up, and everyone there really cares how you do. For them, your success validates their sacrifices, their hopes and prayers for you. They see your degree almost like it is their degree.

This was always in the back of my mind. I would often find myself worrying about failing and placed a lot of pressure on myself to do well. Everyone had given me so much. I could not fail. I had to honor their support. I think it was this extra pressure that really helped me to succeed as well as I did.

I studied all the time that first year. And with my work schedule, I had no time for myself and was barely getting any sleep at all. I was exhausted all the time, honestly, I don't remember much. But by the end of that year, the work I had put in began to pay off. I really started feeling comfortable with my classes and had made more strides in English, both as a language and in understanding and participating in the culture. And with that new comfort level, it seemed like I had gained some new breathing room in my mind. And with that space came understanding. I started noticing the systems around me, how relationships functioned in this country, how the community was organized, what people were worried about and why, what they were excited about. Suddenly, these things began to make sense to me in a way they never had before, and it was as if blinders had been lifted from my eyes. I no longer felt like an outsider in a strange land. I began to love this place called the U.S. I began to feel an affection for its people, and even saw myself as one of them.

I knew it was time to increase my involvement in this place I now called home. It was no longer enough just to study and excel academically, I had to be a part of the fabric of what was going on around me. So, in my second year of medical school, I focused on getting more involved and giving back.

I started on campus. First, I became class treasurer and took an active role in the Cultural Integrity Committee. I was nervous at first, but was surprised how comfortable I felt once I had stepped into those roles. I was able to work well with my peers and took on more and more responsibilities. I met lots of people, and the campus began to feel like a smaller place, a family of people all moving toward the same goals. Pretty soon, professors were mentioning my name and first-year students were coming up to me between classes, asking me how they could get involved in some of the initiatives I was a part of. That was a good feeling, but up to that point, I was only really getting involved on campus. I had a craving to get out there and try to solve real needs in the community around me.

I remembered back to my experiences with the Mercy Ships, how they searched out those that needed help the most, and I started participating in programs to help the underserved communities of rural West Virginia. It was an eye-opening experience for me. Growing up in Cameroon, I always had an image of the U.S. as being this place where everyone is wealthy and none lack, but that was not the truth. I was shocked at what the reality was. There were so many people, particularly in the very rural areas that needed so much. In signing up for some of the programs available, I came in contact with these people regularly.

I started receiving recognition then for my efforts in these programs. The school decided to put my picture up on the front page of the school website. To be honest, I thought they had just done that to show off the diversity of their program, but soon, more and more students were coming up to me asking how they could participate. That's when it hit me. The true impact of being on the website was that others were drawn to this desire to do good in the community. I was all for that.

But with the increased level of notoriety I was receiving, even my friends began to notice. They started playfully calling me Posterchild, and the name eventually spread throughout the medical program.

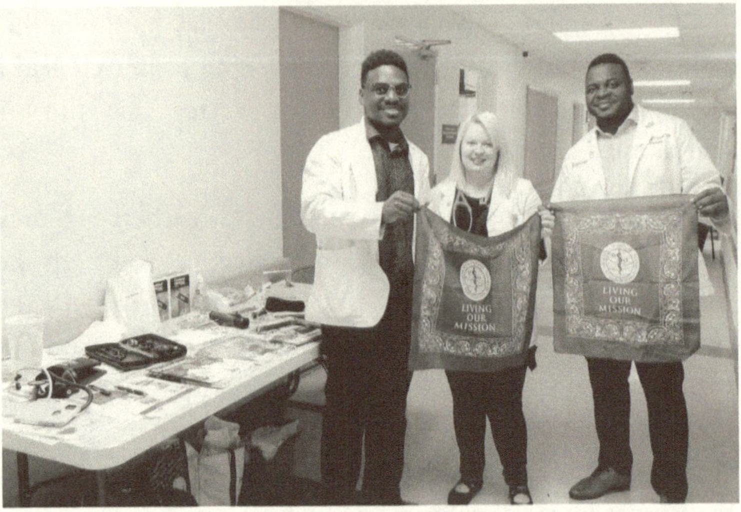

The spark that ignited a movement. One of the first health screenings of The Body Screening Project at Grant Memorial Hospital in Petersburg, West Virginia. This image marks a pivotal beginning, the launch of a health movement driven by a vision to bring essential medical care to those who need it most. It represents the courage to initiate change and the belief in the power of grassroots efforts to transform communities. From left to right, myself, Allison Daniel, my brother, Wilfried Tito.

Serving the underserved became a great passion of mine, so during my third year, I got even more involved. I started participating in the Rural Health Initiative, a program that increases access to quality healthcare in rural communities. It also focused on local high schools, serving as an information and advocacy resource to help local students pursue an education in medicine. During that time, I also joined the Area Higher Education Commission and the Rural Health Association. Even though I still had a full course load and wage-earning work on top of that, I found myself volunteering all of my free time. During my time at the Rural Health Initiative, I learned that, similar to the situation back home in Douala, there weren't enough doctors in the rural areas of West Virginia, and because of that, not enough preventative screening was available to the population. So, in my fourth year, I created a program aimed specifically at that need—a student led initiative called the Body Screening Project.

Every first Saturday of the month, I would go to a local hospital. I would spend the entire day checking vital signs, respiration rates, blood sugar levels. We would give patients full health screenings and provide them counseling about disease related risk factors and health maintenance and preventative behaviors. We taught them about things like diabetes and hypertension and how to avoid these diseases or manage their symptoms.

The program quickly took off. When I started, it was just a thing I did by myself at a local hospital, but pretty soon, the spark had grown into a fire which spread through the community that I was serving. I no longer had the ability to meet the demand alone. I needed help and knew exactly where to look for it. I took the challenge back to my classmates, and it was amazing how ready they were to get involved. All they needed was to see the example and be led. Pretty soon, we had more help than we needed, but the word continued to spread. Neighboring communities asked us to set up similar operations at their hospitals, and what had begun as single town, expanded throughout the county, and then to neighboring counties. . These were all small communities, and the reception was incredible. Everyone knew about us, and everyone was so thankful that we were coming to give them this most important aid. Doctorsfrom other hospitals provided oversight, coming to check in on us and we began forming great relationships with them which stretched back to the university and its programs.

The organization continued to grow, and soon we had so many people willing to help that we had to look for more places to help at. We were even able to attract volunteer medical students from other schools. We started going to nursing homes, showing up at local events, festivals, community gardens, anywhere we thought we would be in contact with people that needed free preventative health care.

Because of my involvement in serving rural communities, I was named the West Virginia Outstanding Student of the year in 2019. I also received a scholarship from the United Health Foundation. And during all this time, I served as the class president for three years.

But even then, it would seem, adversity was not yet done with me. At a time when everything was going well and I felt the closest I had felt to being right where I wanted to be in my pursuit of medicine, I learned that I had failed the COMLEX (Comprehensive Osteopathic Medical Licensing Examinations) seven months before I graduated medical school. I couldn't believe it. It was like something from a dream, a nightmare. I was excelling in all of my classes. I was confident in the material. I simply couldn't believe that I was fail yet another major exam. All I could think about was the MCAT—the very first thing that had prevented me from entering medical school.

The exam results were pretty limited. It only said that I had failed and indicated that I had also failed the "humanistic portion" of the test. That hurt more than anything and sent me into a bit of a depression. If there was one thing I always believed I was naturally competent in, it was interacting well with patients and determining the best course of action for their care. In fact, the humanistic portion was actually my highest scoring section during standardized patient practice in the program. How could I have failed it?

I spent miserable days and sleepless nights thinking about that licensing exam and what I could have done differently. But the harsh reality was staring me in the face; it didn't matter what I could have done differently, I hadn't. And the true result of it all was, I was going to have a harder time finding a residency program to further my education. First, though, I was going to have to retake the exam.

I tried finding resources to help me better prepare, but nothing I found was helpful. Ultimately, I went to my mentor and the Dean of the school and learned about a prep class that I could enroll in through the school.

The prep class was fast and difficult. In only two weeks it was like starting over from scratch. I had to retake the practice standardized exams as a part of preparation for retaking the COMLEX.

Everyone I knew was shocked. How could Poster Child have failed the COMLEX? How could Dimi be in a prep class? How could this man who had started a rural community health program need to be going through this?

I remember reaching out to a local church and asking for them to say prayers for me. I called my family and friends back home and asked for the same. Two weeks later, I retook the COMLEX and passed. I can not remember any moment of greater relief in my entire life. I truly believe God was testing me. I believe he was refining my resolve and strengthening my belief in what I was doing, and why.

After the difficulty of getting through the COMLEX I was even more motivated to see the Body Screening Project grow. I spent more and more time recruiting classmates and expanding to reach as many people within the underserved communities as possible.

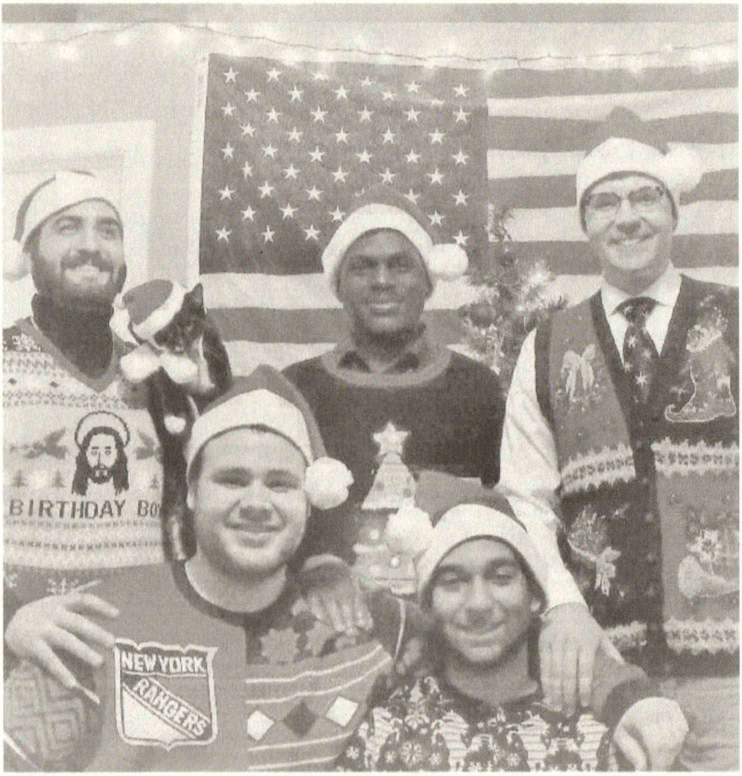

Christmas attire, holiday cards, medical school hustle – a blend of tradition and dedication on the path to purpose. From left to right, Ryan Naum, Vincent Kaykaty, myself, Ameer Quadri, Keaton Dubois.

As I was growing this program, I thought a lot about the people of the Mercy Ships back in Cameroon. That's where it had all started for me, this spark that grew into a fire for helping people. I thought about how all of the doctors on Mercy Ships had jobs elsewhere in the world. These were all doctors in the heights of their careers. They had families and responsibilities like everyone else. They had their home countries that they no doubt missed, and they no doubt had pride for those places. And yet, they had something else. They had a passion for helping people. They had a gaze that sought those who needed help and would not stop at the edge of their responsibilities, or at the border of their familiar world. They allowed it to see further, across cultural barriers, across the globe, wherever the need was greatest.

We have all had our Mercy Ships in life, those caring saviors who came to us just as the need was greatest. None of us got to where we are today, no matter where that is, without the help of others. For some of us, it was our communities that stepped up. For others, it was our family, or even a stranger who happened to lend us a hand. We have all had help. But we also, each one of us, have gifts. We may have money, time, knowledge. We may have a great compassion for a particular community of people in need. We may be able to relate to a certain challenge that a group of others face, perhaps one we too faced or still do. Whatever your gift is, I want to challenge anyone reading this to use it, to step out there, across the borders. Find that person, or group, or community that you can help. You won't be perfect at it; no one ever has been. In fact, you may fail a few tests along the way. You will make mistakes, and that's okay. You don't need to be perfect; you just have to be there. You just have to find that spark in yourself and use it to light the fire around you. Others will see it. Others will come and help fan the flames. And when it is all said and done, you'll be able to look around, and instead of seeing nameless faces going about on unconnected errands—you'll see family.

As for me, I've joined the Army Reserves while I finish my medical training. That's going to give me an opportunity to serve at the local VA hospital and pay back some of my tuition at the same time. I'm still in medical school. I'm still volunteering in rural communities; that's my passion, my spark. That's how I want to give back. I want to become a rural physician who specializes in providing care to small communities. I've taken them on. They are my family now, and my family is growing. Who is your family going to be?

6

BECOMING THE DOCTOR I WAS MEANT TO BE

Graduating from medical school was one of the proudest moments of my life. I still remember that day so clearly—my mother and father sitting in the audience, beaming with pride. My siblings were there too, and the atmosphere was filled with joy, disbelief, and awe. I was the first doctor in my family. Not only that—I was the first to do it overseas, in the United States, far from the place I once called home. To have made it through that journey, arriving in America without knowing a single word of English, and then graduating from one of the top medical schools in the country—it still feels surreal.

Shortly after, I took another step that made me proud: I joined the U.S. Army Reserve. That decision felt like both an honor and a responsibility. But the next professional milestone was residency. I chose Western Michigan University Homer Stryker M.D. School of Medicine to specialize in internal medicine. The move to Michigan was a new chapter —and it started with a funny misunderstanding. I remember seeing the name "Kalamazoo" on the offer letter and thinking it must be somewhere outside the U.S.—Asia or maybe Africa. It just didn't sound American to me. But Kalamazoo turned out to be a small, vibrant city, about 50,000 people, very much part of Michigan and the heart of my next three years.

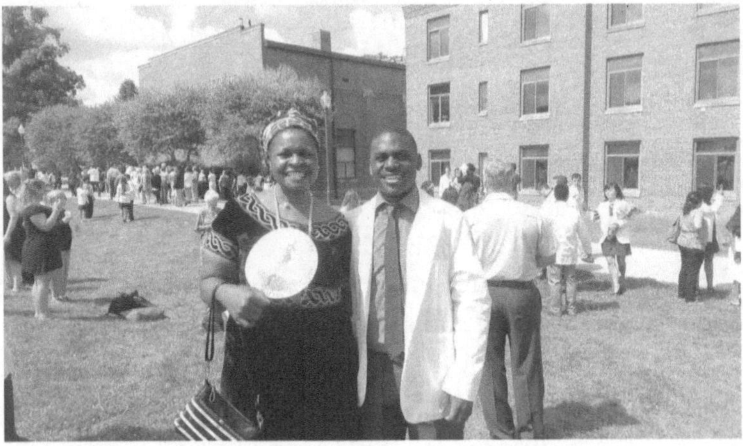

A moment of profound pride and shared accomplishment. Standing with my mother after the white coat ceremony, I was reminded of her unwavering support throughout my journey. She was there at my undergraduate graduation, and here she is again, a constant source of strength and belief as I take this significant step into the world of medicine. This image is a tribute to the power of familial love and its essential role in shaping a physician's path to purpose.

Orientation kicked off in July 2020. I got myself settled in—found an apartment, moved in, and prepared to begin my life as a resident physician. The hospital introduced us to the routines, the departments, and the expectations. To my surprise, residency didn't feel as overwhelming as I expected. I had anticipated chaos and exhaustion, the pressure to prove myself every day. And yes, there was pressure. But I also found it easier than expected to connect—with the other residents, with the staff, and most importantly, with the patients.

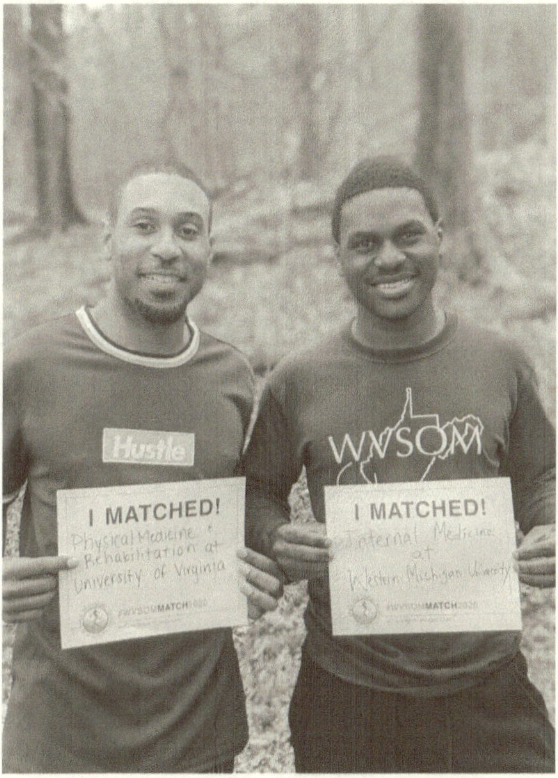

A moment that encapsulates years of relentless effort and unwavering determination. Matching into residency wasn't just a personal achievement; it was the realization of a long-held dream, a pivotal step on the path to becoming a physician. This image speaks to the feeling of accomplishment and the exciting anticipation of the challenges and rewards that lie ahead. Me and Justin Gee. We were the only 2 black male medical students from our class of 2020.

The first year of residency is often considered the hardest. You've got an M.D. behind your name, but you've never really practiced medicine. Suddenly, you're expected to do everything: talk to patients, recognize and treat illnesses, build plans, manage cases, and talk to family members about life-altering conditions. And truthfully, no one cuts you slack. Everyone knows you're new—the nurses, the attendings, the senior residents. Respect has to be earned, not assumed.

But I adjusted quickly. I threw myself into the work. My daily routine was grueling—hospital rounds, patient charts, case discussions, and constant studying—but I kept going. I had this fire inside me, a refusal to give up, a promise to myself that I would become the best doctor I could be. Residency wasn't going to break me. In fact, it became a forge where I was shaped.

By second year, things had changed. I was no longer the nervous new guy. People began to recognize my drive and commitment. I wanted to do more—research, write, attend conferences. I was so committed that my co-residents started joking, saying, "Tito spends more time at conferences than he does in the hospital." I didn't take offense. I knew they saw the ambition behind it. I was learning constantly—about new treatments, new technologies, new research. I wanted to expand my world beyond the hospital walls.

Some faculty encouraged that, but others were more traditional. A few questioned my desire to network or pursue non-clinical opportunities. "Focus on your clinical work," they'd say. "You'll be a better doctor for it." But I wasn't the kind of resident who stayed in the box. I was exploring, pushing boundaries, and seeking mentors who saw beyond the walls of the hospital.

My third year was the turning point. That's when residents start thinking seriously about the future—fellowships, jobs, subspecialties. For me, it was the year I solidified who I was as a physician. I wasn't just a student anymore. I was becoming the doctor I wanted to be. But that transformation came with challenges.

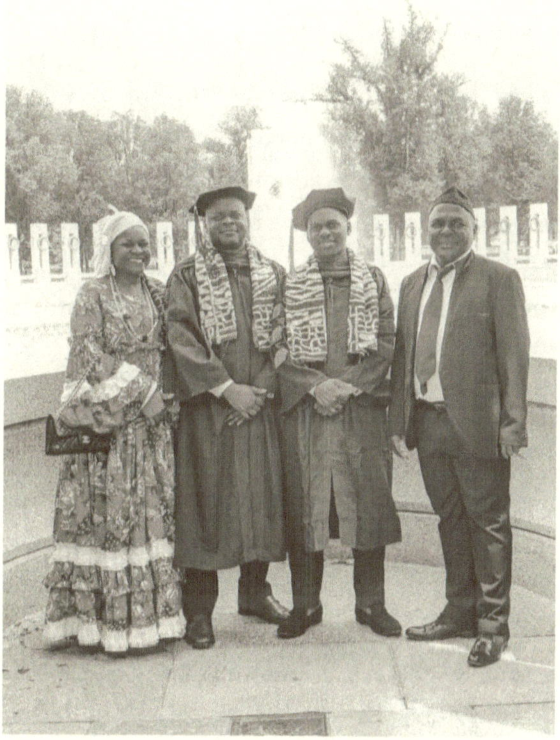

Double the doctors, double the joy! Celebrating a pivotal milestone with my brother, our parents by our side, whose sacrifices and belief paved the way for this dream. This isn't just a graduation; it's a testament to family, perseverance, and the shared pursuit of a calling that now ignites our purpose.

Bias and microaggressions showed up more than I had expected. Yes, I had faced these before—in medical school and elsewhere—but in residency, they took on new forms. Sometimes it was subtle: a nurse questioning a medication I'd ordered, or suggesting I wait on removing a Foley catheter, as if my judgment couldn't be trusted. Sometimes it felt like outright doubt. Orders would be questioned, plans second-guessed—especially when I, a Black doctor in training with an accent, made them.

I remember how painful it was at times. A part of me expected it, but that didn't make it easier. My accent seemed to work against me. In a predominantly white hospital, it was assumed that I must have gone to medical school somewhere else, that I must be new to American medicine. People assumed incompetence without knowing anything about my background, training, or work ethic.

But even in the face of doubt, I stayed steady. I knew that proving myself wouldn't be immediate—but it would be inevitable. My values were my anchor. Much of that came from my time in West Virginia, where I first experienced the culture of close-knit community. People there supported me deeply—church members prayed for me, brought me food during exam weeks, and reminded me that I wasn't alone. That value system, that belief in service and family and connection—it carried me through the hardest days of residency.

And then came the patient who would change everything.

She was 54, the same age as my mother. African-American. Her medical record was one of the most complex I had ever seen—pages upon pages of diagnoses and medications.

Lupus. Diabetes. Hypertension. High cholesterol. Peripheral arterial disease. A whole web of interlocking chronic illnesses. I met her for the first time as a first-year resident, when she came in for an urgent appointment. It wasn't supposed to be anything more than a basic check-in and medication refill. But she was in pain—severe abdominal pain, nausea, vomiting, and rectal discharge. This was no routine visit.

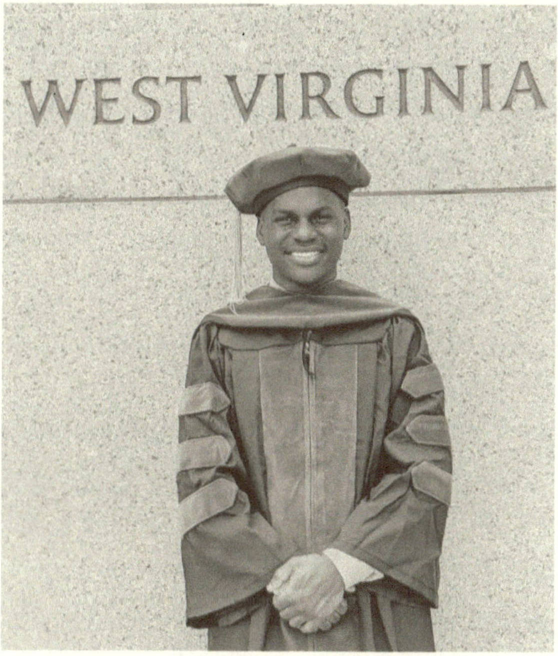

The weight of the gown, the lightness of a dream fulfilled. Wearing my graduation gown after graduating medical school is more than just a photograph; it's a symbol of years of relentless pursuit, late nights, and an unwavering commitment to the calling of medicine. This image captures the profound sense of accomplishment and the hopeful anticipation of the journey ahead, a visual testament to the dedication required to reach this significant milestone and the purpose that now guides my path.

She didn't care that I was new. She didn't care that I was still learning. She needed help, and she needed it now.

Her chart was overwhelming—lab work, imaging, consults from other hospitals across Michigan. I felt the pressure. But I also felt a responsibility. She had prayed that morning that her doctor would figure out what was wrong. And I was that doctor. I had to listen. I had to investigate. I had to act.

We ordered imaging—a CT scan of the abdomen. I gave her medications to ease the symptoms. I consulted with senior residents and attending physicians to make sure I wasn't missing anything. What we found was serious: diverticulitis, an abscess, and a fistula connecting her bowel to her skin—explaining the rectal discharge. It was an advanced complication, and she needed hospitalization and aggressive treatment.

But what stayed with me wasn't just the medicine. It was her trust. Her vulnerability. Her resilience. She reminded me of my mother—not just in age, but in spirit. Despite all she'd been through, she kept showing up. She followed every treatment, took every pill, kept every appointment. And yet, no one had truly listened to her until now.

I gave her my cell phone. I wanted her to feel supported. She called when she couldn't reach the clinic. She texted when she needed refills. And I always responded. Because I understood that her complexity wasn't just medical. It was human. She was exhausted, not just from her illnesses, but from being ignored.

Over time, we built a relationship that lasted all three years of my residency. I became her doctor, and she became like a mother to me. When I graduated, she brought me gifts. She always asked about my wife, about my family. She knew my heart—and I knew hers. That relationship taught me more than any textbook ever could.

I learned that being a doctor isn't about having all the answers. It's about being present. Listening. Caring. It's about recognizing that every patient is a whole person, not just a case file. And if you don't know something, you ask. You seek help. But you never ignore the human in front of you.

That patient—and that experience—helped shape the doctor I am today. A doctor who cares for the underserved. Who listens. Who shows up. And who never forgets where he came from.

Because it's not brilliance that makes a great physician.

It's compassion.

7

WHY I CHOSE INTERNAL MEDICINE

As I REFLECT on my path through medicine, one of the most formative decisions I ever made was choosing internal medicine as my specialty. It wasn't a choice I made lightly—but it also wasn't one I made with full knowledge of every option. The truth is, as a medical student, my exposure was limited. I didn't come from a family of physicians. I didn't have a cousin in orthopedics or an aunt in dermatology to guide me. I only knew the more "visible" specialties—emergency medicine, family medicine, internal medicine, pediatrics, and maybe radiology. That was it.

Looking back now, it's astonishing how little I actually knew about the full landscape of medical specialties. You would think that by the time you're a medical student, you'd have a panoramic view of the field. But for students like me—first-generation physicians from underserved communities—that simply isn't the case. I only discovered some of the more specialized fields after I had already started my residency.

During medical school in West Virginia, most of the physicians I encountered were family medicine doctors working in rural, underserved communities. That was the model I saw again and again—generalists taking care of entire families across generations, managing everything from diabetes to depression. In Lewisburg, where I studied, the focus was always on primary care. The town was small. The needs were great. The doctors wore many hats.

Because of that environment, and my own background, I naturally gravitated toward primary care. I liked the idea of knowing a little bit about everything. I liked the continuity of care, the long-term relationships with patients. I found myself drawn to every specialty I rotated through—surgery, pediatrics, internal medicine. But rather than that being a point of confusion, it actually clarified something for me.

I realized I didn't want to be boxed into one narrow area. I didn't want to only do procedures or only work with children. I wanted the whole picture. Internal medicine offered that. It was the field that allowed me to keep my curiosity broad and my skills diverse. It blended complexity with connection. You had to think deeply, learn constantly, and communicate compassionately. It felt like the perfect fit.

But it wasn't just about what I liked. It was also about who I was becoming. Internal medicine gave me the opportunity to form real relationships with patients. To talk to them, to know them, to walk with them through both chronic and acute conditions. It offered the intellectual rigor I craved while still centering human connection. I didn't want to just treat the body—I wanted to understand the person.

I also have to credit my mentors for guiding me toward that path. Before medical school, mentors were hard to come by. In undergrad, I felt overlooked. There were moments I sensed I didn't belong—bias, microaggressions, a lack of understanding. I didn't have the connections or advantages that some of my peers did. I didn't know how to navigate the system.

But in medical school, things changed. One of my earliest and most meaningful mentors was my clinical skills professor, Dr. Nazar. She believed in me from the start. I remember when I launched the Body Screening Project—a community health initiative to provide free screenings in Petersburg, West Virginia—she was the one who signed off on it. She helped me refine the idea, guided me through the grant application process, and wrote recommendation letters to get us funding. She helped me see that I had something valuable to offer.

She also encouraged me to pursue internal medicine. She said I had the heart and the skill to build real relationships with patients, and that this field would allow me to do exactly that. She saw what I was too young to articulate: that internal medicine would become a foundation not just for my career, but for my mission.

That mission carried into residency. In Kalamazoo, I was fortunate to meet Dr. Baker, another mentor who saw more in me than I saw in myself. I still remember our first conversation during the interview process. She looked me in the eye and said, "If you come here, I will help you. I'll help you become the leader you want to be. I'll connect you with people nationally. I'll support your vision." And she did.

Through her, I was introduced to academic councils, professional organizations, and leadership programs that helped me grow both clinically and personally.

By my third year, I had become the kind of resident others noticed. I was named Resident of the Year—not because I was the smartest, but because I was committed to the work, the people, and the purpose. And that was largely thanks to Dr. Baker's mentorship and belief in me.

There was also Dr. Loehrke, another mentor who left an indelible mark on me. He brought joy to medicine—pure, unfiltered enthusiasm. Every morning, he showed up smiling, energized, and eager to teach. He taught me that how you enter a room matters. That your attitude sets the tone not just for the day, but for the people around you. That energy was contagious, and I carry that lesson with me today when I teach medical students and residents. I want them to feel that same joy, that same purpose. I want them to see that medicine is more than duty—it's a calling.

Of course, my commitment to serving underserved populations started long before medical school. It began in Cameroon, where I grew up witnessing the devastating consequences of medical inequity. I saw people die for lack of three pills. Families broken by the absence of antibiotics. Children orphaned because their parents couldn't afford basic care. And those were the lucky ones. Some lived too far from any clinic or hospital to even get the chance.

That injustice stayed with me. When I arrived in the U.S., I saw different versions of the same story—especially in Appalachia. In West Virginia, many patients didn't have insurance or didn't qualify for Medicaid. Others lived hours from the nearest clinic or couldn't pay the co-pays even when they were insured. Transportation, housing instability, food insecurity—these were the real issues beneath their medical diagnoses.

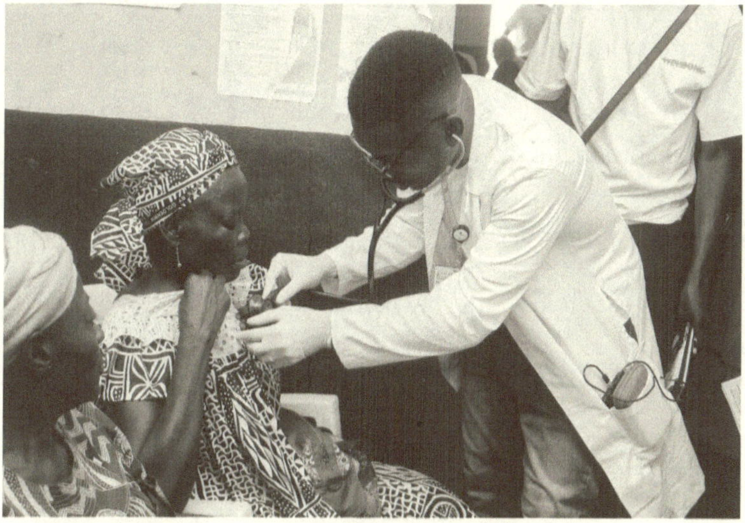

A moment of connection, a commitment to care. Examining a patient at New-Bell Protestant Hospital during our 2024 Annual Health Screening Campaign. This image embodies the essence of direct patient care, the importance of empathy, and the dedication to providing thorough medical evaluations. It's a reminder that at the heart of every health screening is a human being deserving of attention and care.

And so, while I trained in bigger cities like Kalamazoo, my mind never strayed far from the smaller towns and forgotten communities I had served. I kept asking myself: What about the people who can't come to the hospital? What about those whose biggest problem isn't their diabetes, but how to get their child to school or put food on the table? What about them?

That question fueled my passion for expanding the nonprofit I had started in West Virginia. The Body Screening Project had to grow. I knew it. I wanted to take it beyond the borders of the U.S., to make it international, to bring free preventive care to the places that needed it most.

That is still my mission.

Internal medicine gave me the tools. My mentors gave me the encouragement. And my own story—of growing up in Cameroon, of struggling through undergrad, of finding purpose in rural West Virginia—gave me the heart.

I didn't just choose internal medicine.

In many ways, it chose me.

8

BECOMING THE ATTENDING

When I think back to the day I officially became an attending physician, the memory is surreal. The transition was smoother than I expected, but it came with a weight I hadn't fully grasped until I stood in those shoes. To be honest, I never thought I'd get there. Not because I didn't believe in myself, but because the title felt so far away when I first began my journey—just a dream floating in the distance. And yet, there I was. A full-fledged attending. A physician. Independent. Trusted. Responsible.

For those outside medicine, becoming an attending means you've completed your residency, passed your board exams—in my case, the American Board of Internal Medicine—and are now allowed to practice medicine on your own. There's no longer a senior resident reviewing your decisions, no attending double-checking your orders. You become the authority. The decisions are yours. The risks, the consequences, the triumphs—yours too.

At first, that realization was daunting. I remember placing my first orders into the electronic medical record and thinking, "No one's coming to verify this." It was just me now. No safety net. No one hovering behind me to catch a dosing error or to remind me to consider a secondary diagnosis. Every choice I made—whether it was starting an IV, adjusting a medication, or preparing for a procedure—would affect someone's life. That was sobering.

In those early days, I triple-checked everything. I reread protocols, double-confirmed doses, and ran through checklists in my head before moving forward. Not because I didn't trust my training—but because I knew the margin for error in medicine is razor-thin. One mistake could cost a life. One oversight could break trust. I knew mistakes were part of being human, but in this field, the stakes were different. We don't get the luxury of trial and error when the consequence is someone's health—or worse, their life.

And yet, even with that pressure, stepping into the attending role gave me something I never had before: authority and autonomy. But perhaps the most surprising part was becoming a teacher.

My first attending role was at none other than the Johns Hopkins School of Medicine. That still feels strange to say out loud. I hadn't expected it. After graduating from residency, I imagined myself working in a small hospital, building up slowly. But life had other plans. I had completed an academic medicine fellowship after residency, a year of extra training that taught me how to thrive in academic institutions—not just clinically, but as a teacher and a leader.

That additional layer of preparation helped me step into my role at Hopkins with confidence.

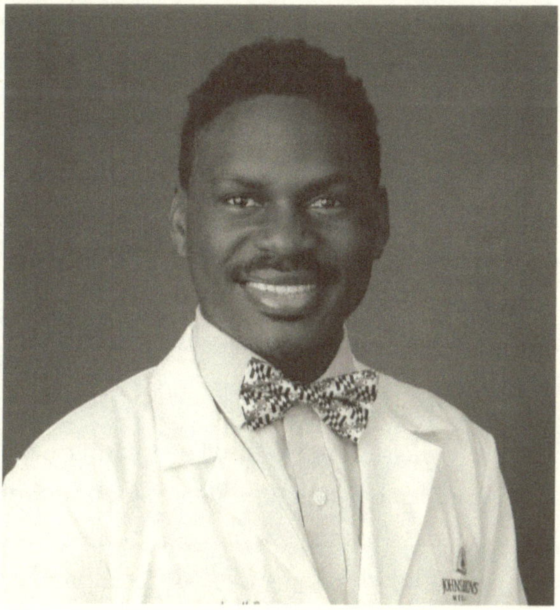

Stepping onto the hallowed grounds of The Johns Hopkins Hospital for the first time as an attending physician. This day wasn't just a career milestone; it was the culmination of years of relentless dedication, sacrifice, and an unwavering commitment to the art and science of healing. A new chapter begins, filled with both immense responsibility and boundless opportunity to make a difference in the lives of others.

My job was twofold. I was an assistant professor and a hospitalist. I spent my days seeing patients, but also training residents and medical students. Teaching clinical skills. Guiding interns on how to speak to patients. Helping them design treatment plans. Watching them navigate uncertainty with the same nervous energy I remembered feeling just a few years prior.

In those teaching moments, I thought a lot about my own education—what I learned and what I didn't. In medical school, I believed that if I was the smartest doctor in the room, that would be enough. I'd be the first to solve a case, the one who cracked the mystery diagnosis. I prided myself on that goal.

But when I became an attending, my perspective shifted. I realized that patients don't just want brilliance. They want to be heard. They want a physician who listens, who understands, who cares. We don't learn that in the textbooks. We don't get tested on empathy or bedside manner. Yet it's one of the most vital parts of being a good doctor.

So I made it my mission to teach what I hadn't been taught. Communication. Emotional intelligence. Conflict resolution. Leadership. Time management. Even health policy—because knowing how systems like Medicare and Medicaid work can make a world of difference in helping our patients navigate the healthcare maze. I wanted to equip my residents with tools that stretched beyond stethoscopes and lab values.

I often shared my own training in health policy with them, explaining how a bill becomes a law, how public health funds are allocated, and why doctors need to have a voice in shaping the systems we work within. Because to truly advocate for patients, we must understand the structures that limit or enable their care.

And even now, just a few years into my attending role, I still see myself as a student. I've only been practicing independently for four years. I'm still learning—still growing. But I continue to equip myself with the skills I need to lead with integrity, purpose, and humility.

A large part of that philosophy was shaped during my time in West Virginia. Those years weren't just a phase—they were a foundation. It was there, in small rural towns, that I learned to ask patients questions no medical exam could reveal. I would ask about their families, their homes, their transportation, their faith. Not as an afterthought, but as a crucial part of their care. Because their struggles—whether political, financial, or spiritual—often dictated their health far more than any lab result.

I began to understand that illness isn't isolated. It lives in a context—a family, a culture, a belief system. And if I didn't ask about those things, I was missing half the diagnosis.

In West Virginia, I learned the importance of meeting people where they were. I remember asking patients how they got to the hospital. Whether they had heat at home. Whether their treatment plan would conflict with their religious beliefs. Whether they had someone to support them through recovery. Those conversations taught me that medicine isn't just about the body—it's about the mind and the spirit too.

That holistic approach stayed with me. It became the core of who I am as a physician. My role as an attending isn't just to treat. It's to teach, to listen, to lead.

I am not here to impress my patients with medical jargon. I am here to hear them.

To see them.

To care for them fully.

And that, above all else, is what becoming an attending has meant to me.

9

WEARING THE UNIFORM - MY JOURNEY INTO THE ARMY RESERVE

Joining the Army Reserve was not something I had planned for when I first began my journey in medicine. But it became one of the most profound and defining decisions of my life. It was born out of a deep sense of gratitude. After everything the United States had given me—the opportunities, the education, the space to grow and thrive—I felt I needed to give something back. Service, to me, was more than a duty; it was a way to express appreciation to the country that had become my second home.

I signed up for the Army Reserve while still in medical school. I chose to enter the medical department of the Army because it aligned naturally with my training and my calling to heal. But even beyond that practical decision, I was driven by a desire to do more—to contribute to something greater than myself, to serve not just patients but the nation.

Of course, there were tangible benefits. The Army helped with tuition, provided a stipend, and assisted with loan repayment. These were not small things. Medical school is financially demanding, and the support offered by the Reserve eased that burden. But my commitment ran deeper than the incentives. I wasn't signing up just for the financial help—I was signing up for the values. For the mission. For the promise to serve.

My perspective on service was also shaped by my time in Appalachia. I often say I "grew up" in West Virginia—not in the literal sense, but in the way that place helped shape my worldview. I was in my early twenties, still impressionable, still figuring out who I was and what I stood for. And what I saw in places like Lewisburg and Petersburg were communities rooted in deep patriotism, despite poverty and struggle. Families there may not have had much, but they had pride. They believed in country, in service, and in each other.

That sense of tight-knit belonging—the familial atmosphere, the honor they placed on military service—left a lasting impression on me. It gave me a renewed understanding of what it meant to be an American and inspired me to embrace that spirit myself. So, I joined not just to repay a debt, but to live out a value system I had come to admire and adopt.

I still remember when the call came for basic training. Boot camp. The real thing. I went through a basic leadership course, followed by medical officer training. As a physician-in-training, my track was slightly different. I was preparing not just to be a soldier, but to be a medical officer—a doctor in uniform. That meant I had to learn the ropes of military life and its unique culture while building on the clinical foundation I had already begun.

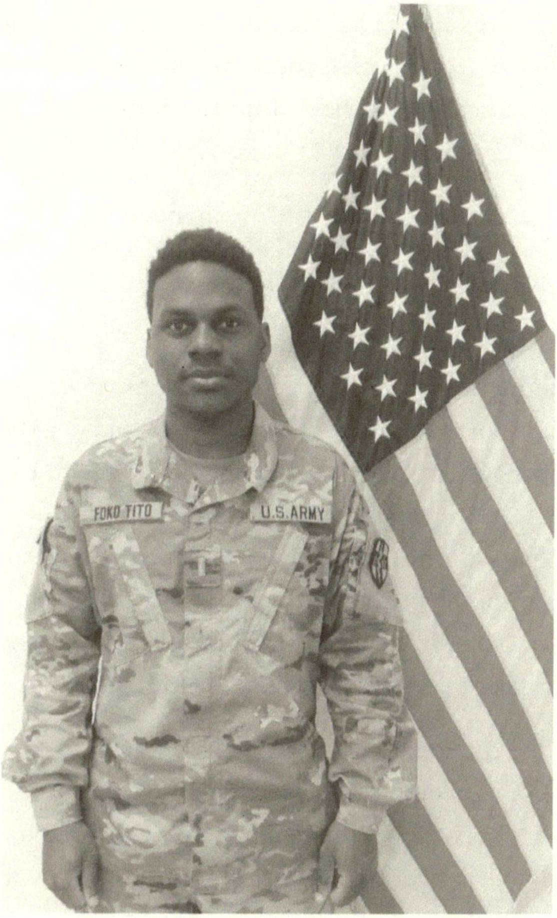

A transformative moment, a commitment to serve. Your first day as a military officer marks a significant transition and a dedication to a higher purpose. This image conveys the pride, challenges, and aspirations that come with embracing this new role, a visual representation of the commitment to service and leadership.

The medical training itself came naturally. After all, I was already immersed in my civilian medical education. Skills like Tactical Combat Casualty Care (TCCC), Combat Lifesaver (CLS), and even Advanced Trauma Life Support

(ATLS) were either familiar to me or close enough in concept that I could pick them up quickly. The IV placements, trauma triage, field injury protocols—I had seen versions of them in my civilian training.

But the hardest part wasn't the medicine.

It was the military itself.

Learning the jargon, the hierarchy, the expectations—it was like entering a parallel universe. Suddenly, I had to understand how to properly address enlisted soldiers versus officers, how to follow the chain of command, how to communicate through formal channels, even how to carry myself in uniform. Things like reporting concerns to the right superior, respecting rank in all situations, and honoring the ritual and rhythm of military life. It was a culture shock—one that demanded both humility and adaptability.

Physically, the demands were steep. Land navigation drills, field training exercises, obstacle courses, and the Army Combat Fitness Test. But coming from Cameroon—where poverty had shaped my resilience—I often joked with fellow trainees that those who grew up poor might actually thrive in the military. The food rations, the limited water, the heat, the manual labor—it felt familiar. Surviving scarcity teaches you discipline. It teaches you endurance. In some ways, the Army was simply another version of what I had already known.

What I hadn't known, however, was the mindset of military medicine. In civilian life, we treat patients with the goal of getting them healthy and comfortable. In the Army, our patients are soldiers—and the goal is different: return them to duty. You're still practicing medicine, but with a different lens. It's mission-focused. It's urgent. It carries a weight that extends beyond the individual.

As a military doctor, you ask yourself: How do I treat this wound so the soldier can rejoin their unit? How do I manage their pain so they can still function in a combat zone? It's a form of medicine that blends healing with readiness. And it took time for me to grasp that distinction.

What struck me most during my training was how tightly woven the fabric of military life really is. The camaraderie. The discipline. The code of ethics. The sense of shared purpose. The military wasn't just another workplace—it was a culture, a family, a way of life. There was no room for shortcuts. Expectations were high. Mistakes carried consequences not just for individuals, but for entire teams, entire missions.

My early days in the Army Reserve taught me about humility, about leadership, and about the kind of doctor—and man—I wanted to be. They reminded me that service isn't always comfortable. It's often demanding, inconvenient, and humbling. But it's also deeply rewarding.

Wearing the uniform gave me a different kind of pride. Not just as a physician, but as an immigrant, as someone who had been welcomed by this country and who now had the chance to give something back—not just in a clinic or a hospital, but on behalf of something much bigger.

Joining the Army Reserve wasn't just an addition to my résumé.

It was an extension of my purpose. A continuation of the values I first learned in Cameroon, nurtured in West Virginia, and now carried forward in every patient I see, in or out of uniform.

10

PREPARING FOR WAR - MY ROAD TO DEPLOYMENT

Deployment was unlike anything I had ever prepared for. Joining the Army Reserve and completing military training had their own challenges—but the moment I was selected for deployment, everything changed. It wasn't just a theoretical possibility anymore. It was real. I was going to war.

It started like any other readiness assessment. I was at Fort Gillem in Georgia attending a Soldier-Focused Readiness Review, or CFIR. These reviews are conducted regularly to ensure that all medical personnel in the Army Reserve are ready—green—for deployment. It's a system of accountability, a way to confirm that every soldier is physically, mentally, and medically prepared to deploy at a moment's notice.

During my last CFIR in 2022, the tone was different. I remember a conversation with my commander, who told me that names were being reviewed for upcoming deployments. Mine was on the list. I'd been in training and academic assignments for years and hadn't been mobilized recently. I assumed, naively, that it might mean another domestic mission—something like the medical support I had previously provided in North Dakota at an IHS facility.

But this time, it wasn't just mobilization.

It was an actual deployment.

To a combat zone.

Northern Iraq.

Near the borders of Syria and Iran.

I still remember the morning it became official. I checked my military email and found a long message: I had been involuntarily selected to deploy. Moments later, my phone began buzzing—calls from my commander, my XO, my unit—confirming that I'd received the notification. Somehow, they knew before I did. They wanted to make sure I understood what was coming.

At first, I was stunned. I'd always accepted the reality of service, but this felt like another world. Iraq. A real combat zone. Active threats. U.S. military targets. Political tensions. The weight of the situation sank in quickly.

To make matters more complicated, I was set to be married that December. My wedding date, venue, and photographer were already booked. Deposits paid. I had envisioned that month as the beginning of a new life, not the start of a deployment. I had to make the painful call to my chain of command and explain. I told them I was prepared to cancel the wedding if needed. I meant it. Service came first. But thankfully, they understood. My deployment was postponed

—just long enough for me to get married and return home for a short time before shipping out.

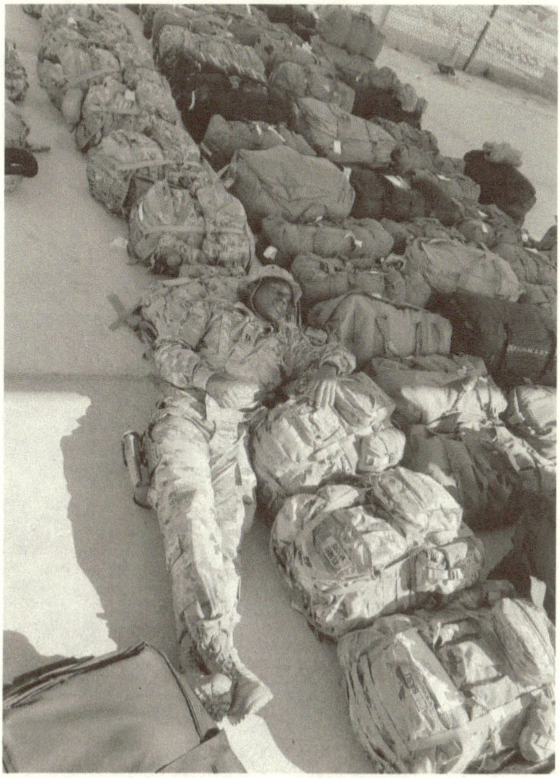

A quiet moment amidst the whirlwind of preparation. In the bag staging area at Fort Sam Houston, prior to deployment to the Middle East, I found a brief respite after an exhausting day as part of the bag detail. This image conveys the dedication, sacrifice, and physical demands of service, while also hinting at the anticipation of the mission and the profound purpose behind the exhaustion.

After the delay, my name remained on the list. I would still deploy. The countdown began.

The preparation for deployment was intense. Physically, mentally, and emotionally. As a medical officer, I had to complete all the standard screenings—Periodic Health Assessments (PHA), dental checks, lab work, vision exams, and mental health evaluations. The Army doesn't take risks when it comes to medical readiness. Everything had to be checked and rechecked. The goal was clear: no surprises overseas.

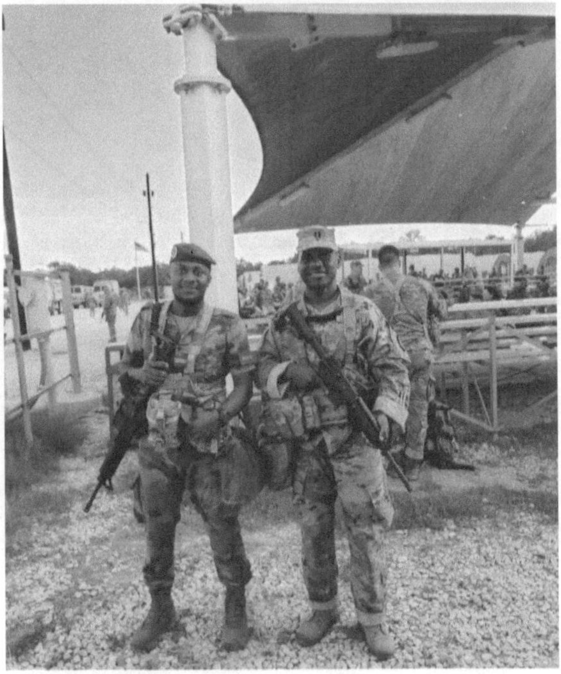

Forging resilience, honing skills. Six months before deployment, engaging in rigorous field training exercises. This image reflects the intense preparation, the physical and mental demands, and the unwavering dedication required of those who serve. It's a testament to the commitment to readiness and the understanding that preparation is key to navigating the challenges that lie ahead.

Training focused heavily on combat medicine. We rehearsed mass casualty scenarios using mannequins and real people. I trained for Role 1, Role 2, and Role 3 facilities—the different levels of care in a combat theater.

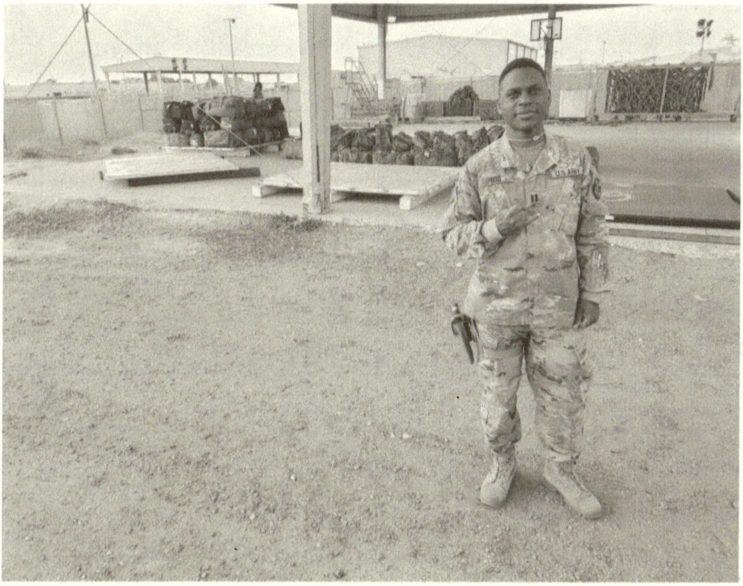

On the cusp of a new chapter, a moment of reflection before the journey begins. This image from Fort Sam Houston, USA, taken prior to our deployment, captures me near the bag staging area – one of my final pictures before heading to the Middle East. It emphasizes preparation, the brink of a journey, and the emotional weight of departure, hinting at the anticipation of what lies ahead.

Role 1 is the first-aid station—immediate triage for wounded soldiers. There, we practiced tourniquets, chest seals, field intubation, shoulder reductions, and quick decision-making under fire.

Role 2 is more advanced—a surgical-capable tent hospital. We learned to perform life-saving procedures like hemorrhage control, minor surgeries, and emergency evacuations. It's limited, but critical for stabilizing patients before transport.

Then came Role 3—the fully functioning field hospital. These facilities are as close to civilian hospitals as possible in a war zone. They include ER sections, ICUs, imaging, radiology, mental health, physical therapy, even a chapel. I trained to operate in the ICU section, managing ventilators, blood transfusions, thoracotomies, and trauma care while under simulated attack. We trained in full gear, during bunker alerts, with sirens blaring. We practiced in dirt, in darkness, in tents, in chaos.

The goal wasn't perfection. It was resilience. We practiced so we could respond automatically—because in war, every second counts.

Emotionally, the contrast between civilian and military life became impossible to ignore. In my civilian job, my day starts with warm coffee, casual conversations, and bedside rounds. I sip my drink, joke with colleagues, call families, play soft music, and write notes in peace. Even on tough days, there's structure, predictability, and comfort.

In the combat zone? None of that exists.

There is no coffee. No slow mornings. No idle chatter about weekend plans. There's dirt. There's urgency. You sleep in a tent—or if you're lucky, a metal container. You wake up at 5 a.m., sometimes earlier, to work out or report directly to the hospital. You're on-call 24/7, treating soldiers injured in blasts or gunfire—or dealing with infections, dehydration, and heatstroke.

There's no routine lunch break. No music. No breaks, really.

You just work.

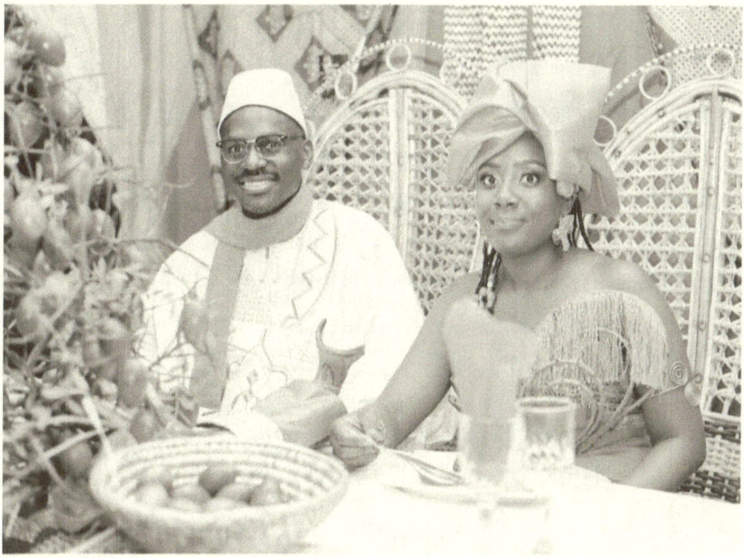

Cameroon, our wedding, Anita. A postponed deployment for love, a new beginning on the journey to purpose.

And yet, what made it even harder wasn't the physical or medical aspect—it was the personal sacrifice. I had just gotten married. My wife and I had just bought a house. I slept there for one night—one night—before I had to leave. I didn't even get a chance to settle in as a husband, to experience the joy of a shared home. We were talking about starting a family, and now, all of that had to be paused.

My wife tried to stay strong. So did my parents and siblings. But deep down, I think they thought I had chosen this. That I had volunteered. That maybe part of me wanted this experience. What they didn't know was how deeply conflicted I felt.

I was proud to serve.

But I was scared too.

Scared to be away for five months. Scared for my safety. Scared of what the deployment might cost me—financially, emotionally, even spiritually. I took a huge pay cut. Army physicians don't earn what civilian hospitalists make. But more than that, I was leaving behind my students, my residents, my co-workers, my family. I had built something at Johns Hopkins. I had built something at home.

And now I had to walk away from it all—temporarily, yes—but with no guarantee of what I would return to.

In those final days before deployment, I found myself clinging to the values I had learned in West Virginia. That place had taught me resilience. It had taught me community, loyalty, and strength in the face of the unknown. I'd seen those values in Appalachia's quiet hills and small towns—families surviving on little, neighbors supporting one another without asking questions. That culture had shaped me. And now, I hoped it would carry me through the months ahead.

I didn't know what Iraq would hold. I didn't know where I'd sleep, who I'd work with, or how safe I would be. I didn't know how I'd feel being away from home, missing birthdays, anniversaries, milestones. But I knew one thing for certain:

I was going.

And I was going prepared—not just with medical skills, but

with purpose, faith, and the belief that service is always bigger than self.

11

LIFE ON THE FRONT LINES – PRACTICING MEDICINE IN IRAQ

When I first stepped foot in Iraq, nothing could have fully prepared me for the experience. I had trained, practiced, drilled, and even imagined what deployment would be like—but still, everything hit differently once I arrived. I was stationed in northern Iraq, near the borders with Syria and Iran, a region steeped in political tension and global complexity.

Even before deploying, my image of Iraq was frozen in time—locked in the early 2000s during the height of the Iraq War. In my mind, I pictured gunfire echoing through crumbling cities, roadside bombs, American soldiers in constant danger, and the looming shadow of terrorist groups controlling entire regions. I knew, rationally, that the official war had ended. But the narrative I had grown up hearing—and the fears echoed by my family and friends—was that Iraq was still a war zone.

Some even confused Iraq with Afghanistan, assuming that the Taliban operated there. They didn't. But the confusion only heightened our collective anxiety. It's hard to unlearn images of war once they're burned into your memory. I braced myself for the worst.

But when I arrived, I was stunned.

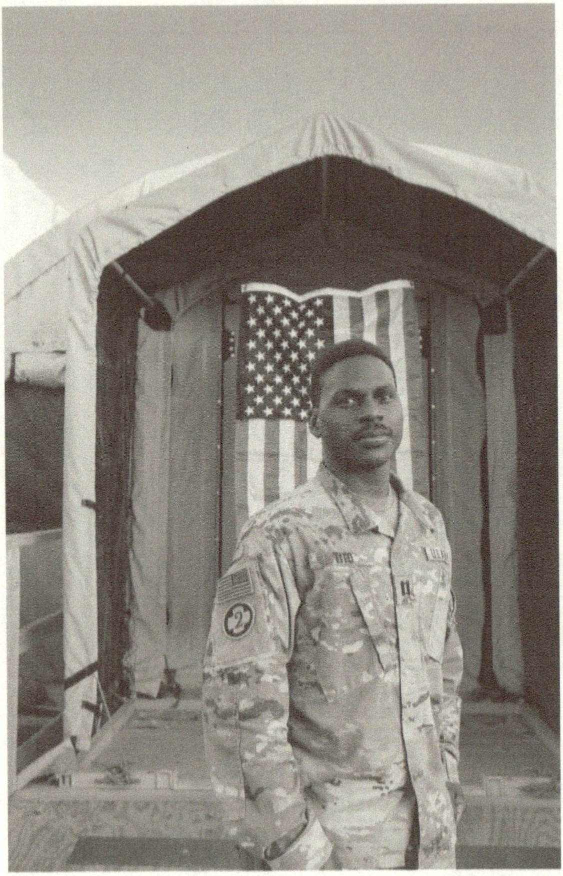

A face shaped by experience, a presence forged in a significant location. This profile image from Iraq captures a moment in time, reflecting the impact of being in a place of profound historical and personal significance. It connects to a specific memory or feeling from that time, a visual reminder of the journey undertaken.

It wasn't the chaos I expected. In fact, the region was calm—almost peaceful in a way that felt surreal. Yes, I was on a military base, and yes, our movement outside the wire was strictly limited. But what I encountered on base wasn't hostility. It was humanity.

The weather was the first surprise. I'd imagined a sun-scorched desert—dry, cracked earth with sweltering heat and camels wandering through dunes. But northern Iraq in winter was something else entirely. The temperature dropped below freezing at night. Mountains rimmed the landscape. It was cold, even icy at times. That visual—snow-dusted terrain instead of an endless desert—shocked me more than anything.

The locals were another revelation. I expected tension, distance, even resentment. After all, we were American soldiers in a land that had experienced war, loss, and division. But the Iraqi civilians who worked on base were kind, generous, and welcoming. They asked about our accommodations, helped us set up our living quarters, and even inquired if we needed anything for comfort. These were men and women who embraced our culture while sharing their own. It was a level of mutual respect I hadn't anticipated.

Our accommodations were modest but manageable. I slept in a "Conex" container that had been retrofitted with heating and basic utilities. Junior soldiers stayed in tents—less insulated, less comfortable, but functional. Access to a generator meant hot water and power, which during those freezing nights, was a small luxury. I was grateful for every bit of it.

The food was... well, forgettable. I had dreamed of Middle Eastern cuisine—spiced meats, fragrant rice, maybe some local flavors. But what we got was pure DFAC: dining facility mass-produced American food. Chicken tenders. Overcooked steak. Rice with no salt. Taco Tuesdays. Mongolian Mondays. Lobster Fridays. It all tasted like cafeteria food made to feed 3,000 people—efficient but uninspired. Still, it filled the stomach.

But what truly redefined my understanding of deployment was the practice of medicine itself.

I had expected constant violence, mass casualties, a nonstop barrage of injuries. Instead, we operated in a state of high readiness—dealing with intermittent trauma, yes, but also supporting ongoing operations in a relatively stable zone. There were moments of intensity—bunker alerts, suspected drone activity, aerial threats—but they came in waves, not an unrelenting flood. The base was forward-positioned, and our field hospital had only recently been established. Much of our mission was to build it up, stabilize it, and prepare it to care for soldiers deployed across the region.

The hospital setup presented its own challenges. In the U.S., hospitals are structured, resourced, and shielded from external noise. In Iraq, our hospital was a tent. The ICU was a tent. The ER was a tent. There were no permanent walls, no private offices, no quiet corners to retreat to. Patients were beds apart, and privacy was almost nonexistent. In a civilian setting, violating HIPAA can get you fired. In combat, maintaining privacy is almost impossible. Even your most sensitive patient encounters—mental health discussions, psychiatric evaluations—happen within earshot of others.

That was hard. We did our best, but the environment didn't allow for perfection.

Then there was the noise. Constant. The thunder of Blackhawks overhead, Chinooks landing, training exercises thudding in the distance, gunfire echoing from ranges, radios buzzing, doors slamming. Practicing medicine under these conditions required a new kind of focus. Procedures that required precision—like placing central lines, intubating, or managing trauma—became acts of extreme concentration.

And the volume of people. There was never a moment alone. The ER was full. The ICU was full. The medical tent was always active. Radiologists—who in civilian life work quietly in dark rooms—had no such privilege here. One of my colleagues, a radiologist, often joked (though not entirely) that reading scans in this environment was the hardest thing he'd ever done.

Still, we adapted. We had to.

We practiced casualty scenarios repeatedly—battle drills, bunker transfers, mass casualty simulations. We planned how to evacuate patients from the hospital to bunkers. Who would carry the medications? Who would manage non-ambulatory patients? Who would stay behind with critically ill soldiers during an incoming threat? We trained for it all.

And then we lived it.

I remember a time when we had an actual bunker alert. Sirens blared. Incoming threat detected. No time to hesitate. We ran—into the hospital, risking ourselves—because patients were there. Some couldn't walk. We helped them, gathered their IV fluids, oxygen tanks, medications, and wheeled them to safety. During one surgical procedure, we faced an alert mid-operation. And we kept going. That's what we signed up for.

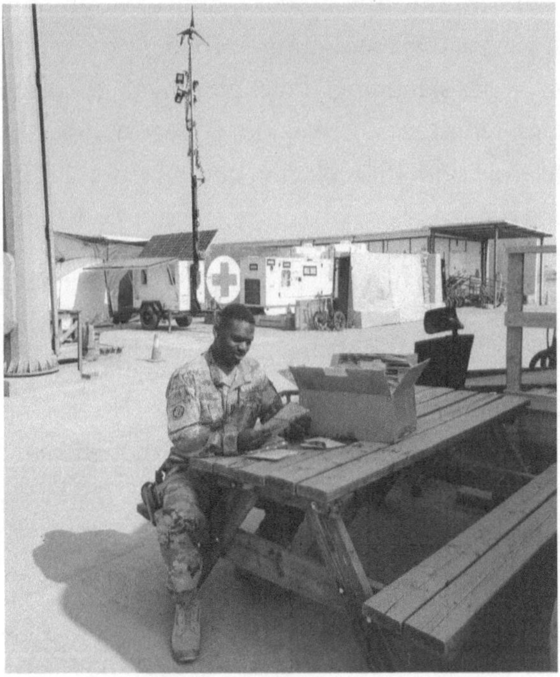

A tangible link to home, a reminder of unwavering support. While serving overseas in Iraq, I received a heartfelt care package from my colleagues at Johns Hopkins Bayview Medical Center. This image captures a moment of opening that package, reading the cards filled with warmth and encouragement. It's a powerful testament to the bonds of camaraderie that transcend distance and the profound impact of knowing you are remembered and supported by those who share your calling. This simple act of kindness fueled my spirit and strengthened my resolve during a challenging time.

The expectations were clear. As medical officers, our mission was not just to heal but to return soldiers to duty whenever possible. We couldn't afford to sideline a soldier for every minor injury. Commanders expected their troops back—quickly, if not immediately. The philosophy had shifted toward large-scale combat readiness. We triaged differently. We weighed functional ability over comfort. Could the soldier perform? If yes, they stayed. If not, they were reassessed—but always with the mission in mind.

Every decision was layered. Medical judgment. Command intent. Soldier readiness. It wasn't easy. It wasn't calm. But it was real.

And through it all, I drew on the same strength I had developed years before in West Virginia. That rural spirit—of resilience, of resourcefulness, of community—showed up in every interaction, every emergency, every difficult moment. The culture of camaraderie I witnessed there felt mirrored here, in a place half a world away, surrounded by sand and tension.

That's what deployment taught me: that medicine is never just about the disease. It's about the moment. The context. The stakes. And sometimes, it's about doing everything you can—with everything you have—in the most unforgiving conditions imaginable.

I didn't just practice medicine in Iraq.

I practiced presence. Purpose. Resolve.

And I'll carry those lessons with me for the rest of my life.

12

BATTLEFIELD MEDICINE: THE REALITY OF COMBAT CARE

There were definitely instances where we treated seriously wounded soldiers—moments that truly reflected the reality of battlefield medicine. I knew going in that our team would be responsible for critically ill service members, not just Americans, but also coalition forces—the French, the British, the Germans—and even Iraqi locals and contractors. As a field hospital operating in a combat zone, we were responsible for everyone. Civilians, contractors, allied troops—it was a large and diverse population under our care.

And while most people think only of gunshot wounds or blast injuries in combat zones, the majority of the cases we saw weren't actually combat-related. In fact, many injuries were accidental or medical in nature. For example, we treated soldiers involved in LMTV rollovers—those massive troop transport trucks. We saw traumatic fractures, arm and leg injuries, even eye trauma from accidents with heavy machinery. During the blistering summer months, heat casualties were common. At the weapons range, we occasionally had accidental discharges resulting in gunshot wounds.

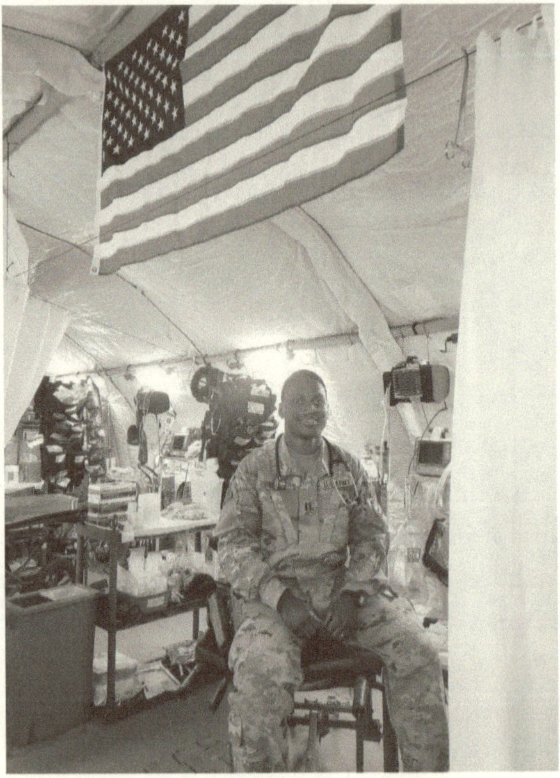

A view of our Field Hospital in Northern Iraq, a beacon of healing amidst the complexities of supporting Operation Inherent Resolve (OIR). This image captures more than just a structure; it represents the dedication, resilience, and unwavering commitment of the medical teams working tirelessly within its walls. It speaks to the critical role of medical support in challenging environments and the profound impact of bringing care and hope to those in need.

Medical issues were also a big part of what we treated. Remember, this wasn't just a young, healthy population.

There were civilians and older contractors on base as well. Some presented with uncontrolled diabetes, hypertension, even signs of cancer. We saw unexplained weight loss, night sweats, and swollen lymph nodes—cases that reminded me more of an internal medicine clinic back home than a war zone.

Of course, trauma cases still came in. We had soldiers injured in action, some with gunshot wounds from the enemy. I'll never forget one soldier who came to us after sustaining a severe neck injury while training Syrian Democratic Forces. He had been air medevac'd from Syria, bleeding profusely when he arrived. We immediately initiated care according to Tactical Combat Casualty Care (TCCC) guidelines. Pressure to stop the bleeding. Large-bore IVs. Blood transfusions. Fluids. Pain control.

I remember looking at him—this infantryman, a guy trained for combat—and seeing something deeper. He wasn't just a soldier. He was a husband. A father-to-be. As he lay there, pale and weak, he prayed to survive, to make it home. It struck me: we tend to think of these guys as unbreakable. But in that moment, he showed me the human side of war.

We stabilized him and got him to surgery. Imaging had revealed a ricocheted fragment lodged in his neck. The trauma surgeons—experts in vascular repair—worked quickly to control the arterial bleed and repair the vessel. It was a team effort. That's what combat medicine demands. When a trauma hits, we activate everything—radiology, lab, pharmacy, surgeons, techs. It takes a full hospital to save a single life, and that's exactly what we did.

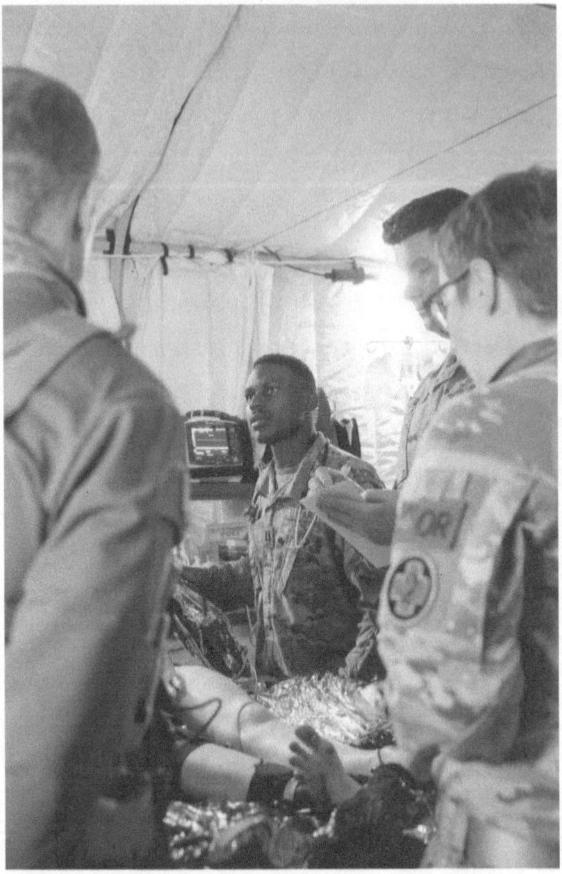

Providing compassionate care with Coalition Forces in an Iraq field hospital – a testament to global cooperation and dedication. MAJ Jane Cowan (Trauma surgeon) and MAJ Emil Gurau (ICU RN) seen on the right side of the image.

Our field hospital was better equipped than many might expect. We had CT scanners, labs for checking blood counts, a pharmacy with IV meds and antibiotics. Despite the pressure and resource limitations, we were able to provide real care. We had other cases that left a mark, too. A civilian contractor presented with signs of advanced cancer. We were able to image him, confirm the diagnosis, and begin supportive care. Not every story had a heroic save, but each reminded me why we were there.

One case that hit especially hard was a suicide attempt by a deployed soldier. It was a gut punch. We're all called to serve, but the stress affects people in different ways. Some cope. Some break. This particular soldier had reached his limit. We found him just in time. Administered reversal agents, IV fluids, supportive care. We stabilized him, but we knew his care wasn't just medical—it was psychological. We got him connected with behavioral health and helped him find healthier ways to cope.

The mental health burden in the combat zone is real. And we didn't just treat injuries—we treated people. Broken bones and broken spirits. Gunshot wounds and grief. Diabetes and depression. It was all part of our mission.

Our team was multidisciplinary—surgeons, radiologists, psychiatrists, pharmacists, ENT, ophthalmology. No, we didn't have every specialty, but we had the essentials. We worked within limitations. For example, we didn't have MRIs, and some labs we would've ordered stateside weren't available. But combat medicine isn't about extensive testing—it's about saving lives. It's about stopping the bleeding, stabilizing the vitals, and returning service members to duty when possible.

We didn't need fancy equipment. What mattered was knowing how to act under pressure. Knowing how to apply a tourniquet correctly. Knowing when to call for blood. Knowing how to intubate with minimal space and maximum noise around you. We trained for it, and we relied on each other.

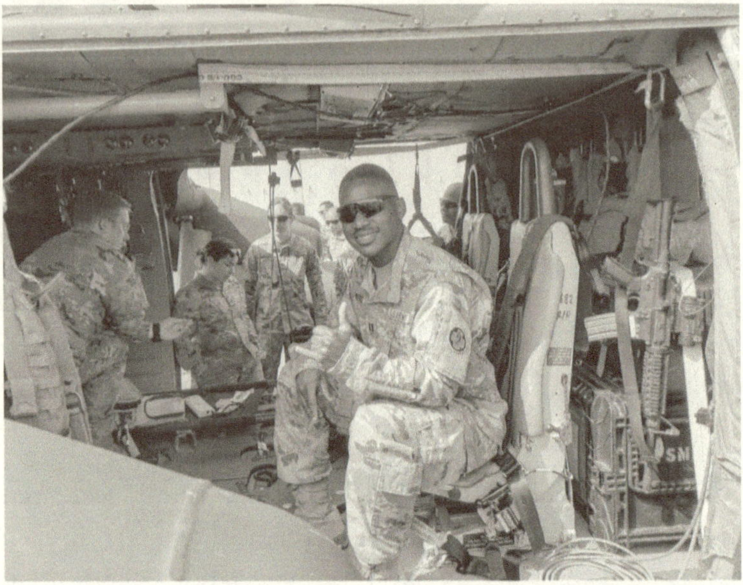

Within the heart of a rescue, a symbol of bravery and immediate impact. Posting in a UH-60 Black Hawk MEDEVAC shortly after a rescue mission, I witnessed the critical service being provided firsthand. This image highlights the courage of those involved and speaks to the feeling of a mission's completion and the lives saved, a powerful reminder of the impact of rapid medical response.

There were moments where we had to run into the hospital during bunker alerts. Incoming drones, suspected missile strikes—we had to move fast. Some patients weren't ambulatory, so we carried them. Grabbed oxygen tanks, meds, IV pumps—whatever they needed. We even had to evacuate the OR mid-surgery during one alert. That's the kind of environment we were working in. You don't pause for coffee. You don't take a break. You keep moving. You adapt.

And in all that chaos, the priority remained the same: treat, stabilize, return to duty. The Army was shifting toward readiness for large-scale combat operations. That meant we couldn't afford to send everyone home for every injury. Minor injuries had to be managed on-site. We had to decide quickly—can this soldier return to duty? Light duty? Or do they need to be evacuated? These weren't just clinical decisions—they were operational ones.

In a civilian hospital, you might have time. You might have privacy. In a field hospital, space is limited. Privacy is nearly impossible. Soldiers are treated side by side. Battle buddies check on each other. Staff are constantly moving in and out. I used to joke about HIPAA—how back home, you'd get fired for a privacy violation. In combat medicine, privacy is a luxury. Still, we did our best. When a case demanded it, we'd find a private area. But most of the time, everyone knew everyone's business.

We made it work. We had to. We didn't need the latest surgical robot or state-of-the-art imaging. We needed skill. Grit. Teamwork. And heart.

That's what combat medicine is. Not perfect. Not pristine. But real. Messy. Urgent. And deeply human.

13

COMBAT MEDICINE REFLECTION

THE HUMAN TOLL of war goes far beyond the physical wounds we treated on the battlefield. It extends deep into the emotional and psychological scars, not just for civilians, but for soldiers as well. During my deployment, I came face-to-face with those realities in ways I hadn't fully anticipated.

One of the most jarring moments for me was discovering how many service members struggled with suicidal thoughts while deployed. I had assumed such mental health crises were confined mostly to the civilian world. I was wrong. War zones don't suppress inner turmoil; they amplify it. The stress, the noise, the fear, the sleep deprivation—it all compounds. The high expectations, the sense of constant danger, and the weight of one's responsibilities can become unbearable. Rockets fired in the distance, the boom of aircraft overhead, and the knowledge that your life is not entirely in your control—it chips away at a person. Some soldiers just couldn't cope, and it pushed them to the brink.

Sleep was a luxury we rarely enjoyed. Nights were filled with constant noise from helicopters or jets landing and taking off from the nearby airstrip. My cot was narrow and uncomfortable, and I often slept only four or five hours a night—sometimes even less if I was called into the hospital for a trauma case. The cumulative exhaustion wore on all of us.

Food was functional, not enjoyable. We ate three times a day, but it wasn't what anyone would call nutritious or comforting. It was meant to keep us alive and moving, not satisfied. On top of that, we were far from our families. While I had the maturity and life experience to handle it, I could see the emotional strain it placed on the younger soldiers, some barely out of high school. Being away from loved ones for nine to twelve months during formative years takes a psychological toll that can't be measured.

There were times I questioned everything. Why had I signed up for this? Why was I in Iraq while my wife was back home, starting a new chapter in her life without me? She had gone back to school for nursing and was struggling through difficult classes on her own. We had just gotten married, bought a new house, and yet I'd only slept in our home once before deploying. My mother had fallen ill and been hospitalized while I was away. I missed her birthday, my wife's birthday, my siblings' graduations, even my best friend's trip with our group of friends. I missed so much. It hurt.

Still, each day I went to work and treated service members, something kept me going. I found meaning in caring for them, helping them heal, and sending them back to duty. I saw them at their most broken and then watched them recover. That gave me a deep sense of purpose. I wasn't carrying a rifle into battle, but I was in the fight—saving lives.

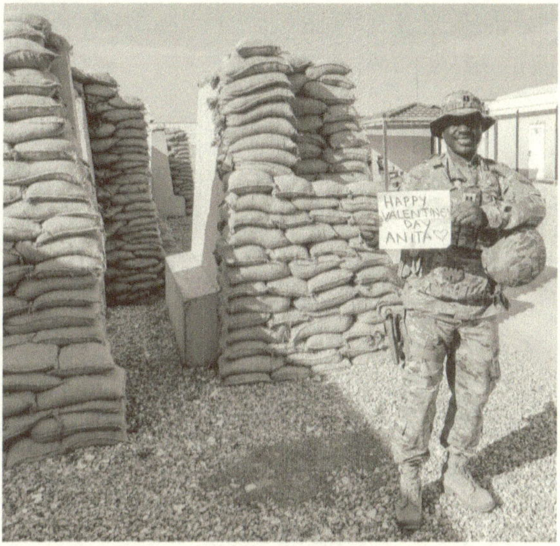

Love knows no boundaries, not even thousands of miles and a war zone. Sending a heartfelt Happy Valentine's Day message to my beloved wife, Anita, from Northern Iraq. This image is a poignant reminder of the personal sacrifices made by those in service and the enduring strength of the bonds that connect us to those we love, offering a beacon of hope amidst the challenges.

Professionally, I left behind a job I loved. I worked at Johns Hopkins with an amazing team. My boss, my colleagues, the trainees—they were more than coworkers; they were like family. We shared lunches, weekends, casual conversations about life. I missed that closeness, that normalcy.

Internet access was limited and monitored, so connecting with home wasn't always easy. And because of the nature of our work and our location, much of what we did couldn't be disclosed. I had to carry the weight of those secrets alone. Living in such close quarters with the same people for so long also had its challenges. While there was camaraderie, there was also conflict. You start to see each other's habits and flaws a little too clearly.

But there were beautiful moments, too. I remember visiting the French compound, where we shared non-alcoholic beers and stories. Being from Cameroon, I spoke French fluently, which allowed me to connect with their team on a deeper level. We discussed life, military service, Africa, and what it meant to be deployed. The same with the Germans. They invited us for waffles on Saturdays—freshly made, topped with Nutella and strawberries. We talked about our medical training, our home countries, our dreams.

The Italians, with their small but incredible pizza restaurant, gave us a taste of home. Their hospitality was unmatched. Even with limited English, we shared laughter, meals, and stories. The Estonians had a spa—yes, a spa—which they claimed was standard in every one of their bases worldwide. They joked often, but were sharp, disciplined, and some of the most reliable people I met.

Even my preconceived notions about the local Iraqi civilians were shattered. They were kind, helpful, and deeply appreciative of our presence. They guided us, taught us their customs, helped us navigate their culture, and even taught me more Arabic than I had learned back in the States. From their cuisine to their music, I was given an intimate view of their lives.

The coalition spirit was powerful. We weren't alone. The British, Italians, Estonians, Germans, French—all of us worked together. When a trauma came through our hospital doors, everyone showed up. It didn't matter the patch on your shoulder. We were one team, with one goal: to save lives.

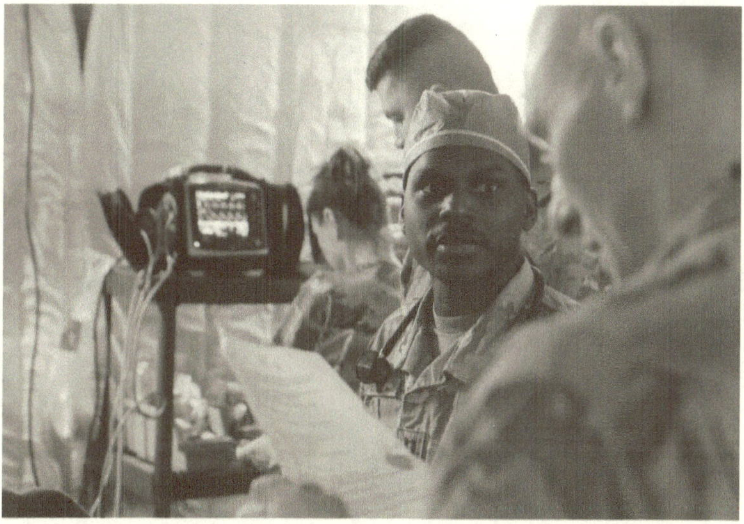

Within the walls of a Mixed Critical Care unit in an Iraq field hospital, every second counts. This is where the stakes are highest, and the demand for medical expertise is paramount. This image is a testament to the resilience of the human spirit and the tireless efforts of the medical teams who navigate complex challenges to provide life-saving care in the most demanding of environments.

That kind of medicine isn't about having the latest technology. It's about trust. It's about skills. It's about being calm under pressure, relying on your training, and leaning on your teammates. Even when resources were limited, we made it work. Even with stress and fear in the background, we delivered care. Because in that place, with so many people depending on us, we didn't have a choice.

Yes, there were moments I was scared. Yes, there were moments I questioned my decisions. But I had faith in my mission. And I knew, without a doubt, that I was not alone.

14

DOCTOR IN A WAR ZONE

SERVING as a doctor in a war zone is ultimately about finding purpose through service. Very few doctors ever deploy to active conflict zones. If less than 1% of the U.S. population serves in the military, the number of physicians who volunteer and are sent into combat zones is even lower—less than 0.5%. Many see physicians as too valuable to risk: their training takes years, and their loss would be profound. There's a fear: what if something happens?

But I knew my role. I was there to build and support a field hospital, to provide care to the wounded, and to return soldiers to duty as quickly and safely as possible. That meant treating everything from battlefield trauma to illnesses, from minor injuries to life-threatening emergencies. And it meant being prepared to stabilize and evacuate patients to higher levels of care—sometimes to Germany, sometimes back to the United States.

Yet beyond the physical care, I also became a source of emotional support. Soldiers didn't just bring in broken bones or burns—they brought in their burdens. They came to talk, to offload the stress of being far from home, the strain of combat, the wear of the unknown. Many of them were dealing with anxiety, depression, and overwhelming loneliness. I often found myself listening more than prescribing. In that listening, I discovered something unexpected: I shared their pain.

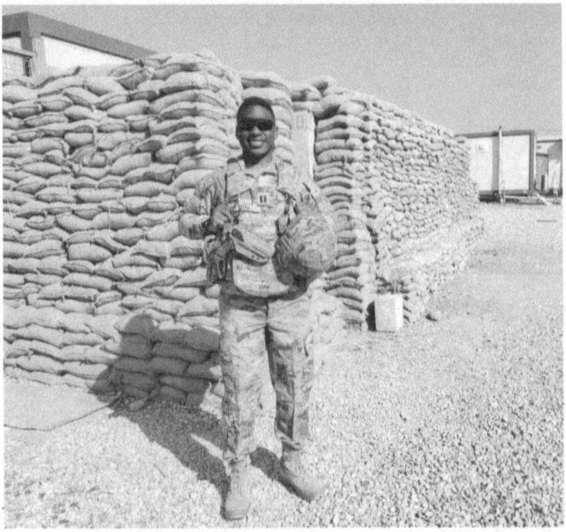

Bringing healing and hope to a critical region. Somewhere in Northern Iraq, I had the opportunity to provide medical support, contributing to Operation Inherent Resolve (OIR). This image highlights the critical humanitarian or military support being offered, and speaks to the profound impact on lives that comes with such dedicated service.

I too was far from home. I too was anxious. I too felt the weight of absence—the absence of my family, of my wife, of the milestones I was missing. But in those moments, I had to set my struggles aside and be present for someone else. That's what made it powerful. On the civilian side, I never truly shared the medical burdens my patients described—I wasn't diabetic or hypertensive; I didn't live with chronic pain. But in Iraq, I finally experienced something in common with my patients. We were both enduring the same emotional landscape, just from different positions in the hospital.

As the weeks passed, my role evolved. Initially, I thought I was just there to treat wounds—to save lives, as I'd seen in movies. But I soon realized my work went deeper. I wasn't just restoring life—I was maintaining it. I became a mentor, a counselor, and a quiet presence for the soldiers and staff around me. I'd talk with the NCOs and enlisted troops about family, purpose, and home. I answered medical questions, yes, but also life questions. Over time, I became a trusted figure—not only as a physician, but as a fellow human being navigating the same terrain.

It reminded me of my time practicing medicine in West Virginia, where listening—really listening—had taught me more about people than any textbook ever could. Soldiers, like patients back home, carried unique stories. Some joined the military out of a sense of duty, continuing a family legacy of service. Others enlisted because they had no other direction. Each reason mattered. Each person mattered. And I shared my story too—how I joined to give back to a country that had given me so much.

One of the most profound moments of my deployment came in the emergency treatment area. A civilian contractor had collapsed while driving. He crashed his vehicle and was found unresponsive, pulseless. The medics brought him to us. They'd already initiated CPR and intubation en route.

We took over, continuing chest compressions, administering medications, doing everything we could.

But after 30 to 40 minutes, there was no response. We had to stop. I had to pronounce him dead.

I had done this before—on the civilian side, in American hospitals—but this was different. This man had come to Iraq to serve, even if not in uniform. He had left his family, just like us. And now he would never go home. I filled out the death paperwork, numb with the weight of what it meant. Not just the death itself, but the distance—his family would hear of it through official channels, miles and hours away from the moment it happened. There would be no bedside goodbye.

That stayed with me. Because it could've been any of us. And it wouldn't take a rocket attack or enemy fire—life happens in war zones, just like anywhere else. We were all vulnerable. We were all far from home.

Even outside the hospital walls, the role of a physician continued. Sometimes, I led health education efforts—how to stay physically and mentally resilient. Sometimes, I sat beside soldiers just to talk. Sometimes, I mentored junior personnel, guided them through life questions they were too afraid to ask anyone else.

I also found unexpected joy. Interactions with coalition partners—the French, Germans, Italians, Estonians—brought camaraderie. We traded stories, shared meals, discussed our countries and cultures. I found comfort in those small moments. Laughter over waffles with Nutella. Jokes about the Estonian spa. Learning Arabic from the local staff who were warm, kind, and far more welcoming than I'd been led to believe. These weren't distractions—they were reminders of our shared humanity.

My time in Iraq taught me that being a physician in combat is not just about emergency medicine or battlefield trauma. It's about presence. It's about humility. It's about being human with other humans in an inhuman place. And it's about service—not just service to country, but service to people. To their stories. To their survival. To their hope.

COMING HOME, COMING FULL CIRCLE

As far as reflections on my journey, the day we got back to the States was filled with immense joy. I remember each stop on the way out of Iraq—Qatar, Kuwait, Germany—and finally, Portsmouth, New Hampshire. That first stop on U.S. soil felt monumental. We stepped off the plane to be greeted by veterans, many from the Vietnam era, and USO personnel welcoming us home. I must have heard "thank you for your service" two dozen times before I even reached baggage claim. It was unexpected and deeply moving.

My battle buddies and I weren't anticipating that kind of reception—especially in a small New Hampshire town. The journey back had taken over 26 hours, zigzagging across the globe with stops to drop off personnel and equipment. It was Army time—not our time. But I was grateful just to be part of it, and even more grateful to be going home.

My wife picked me up from the airport on May 3rd. My birthday had passed just two days before. She greeted me with balloons and joy, and I felt an overwhelming sense of relief and happiness just to see her again. What was supposed to be a three-month deployment had turned into nearly six. That reunion felt sacred.

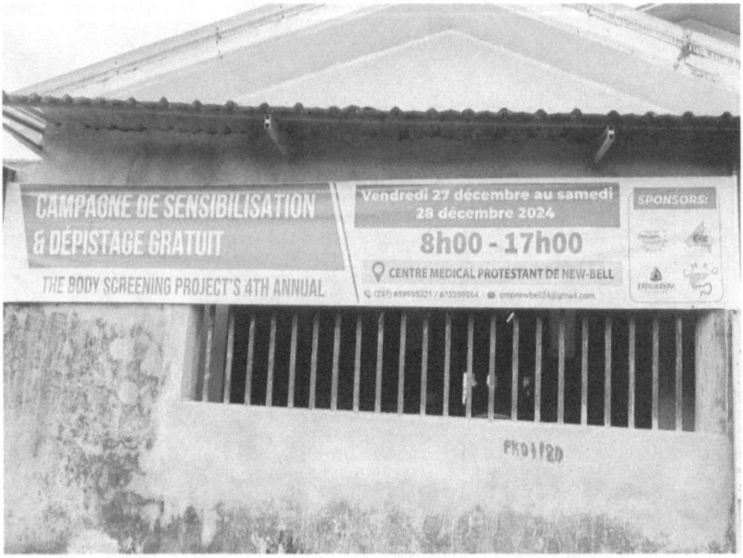

A beacon of hope in Douala, Cameroon. New-Bell Protestant Hospital, the vital location where The Body Screening Project conducted their 2024 Annual Health Screening Campaign. This image provides context for a significant humanitarian effort, highlighting the hospital's crucial role in enabling access to free medical care for the community. It represents the partnership between charitable initiatives and local institutions to create lasting impact.

The next day, we had dinner with my family. My parents and siblings came by to see me. They all had comments: that I'd lost weight, that I looked different, that I seemed more muscular. Deployment has a way of physically transforming a person—but the deeper change was internal.

Driving home from the airport, I found myself staring out the window, overwhelmed by the green—trees, forests, grass.

After months of beige desert, the sight of vibrant vegetation brought tears to my eyes. I noticed the quiet too. No loudspeakers, no alerts, no bunkmates. Just silence. Stillness. Privacy. Home.

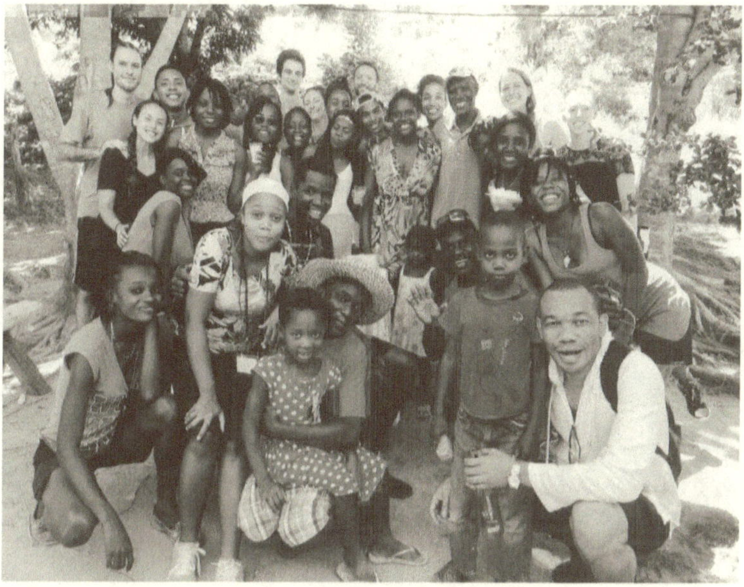

A moment of profound human connection, a commitment to care. Examining a patient at New-Bell Protestant Hospital during our 2025 Annual Health Screening Campaign, I witnessed the direct impact of community service and compassionate medical care. This image embodies the essence of healing, and serves as a reminder that at the heart of every health screening is a human being deserving of attention and care.

Back at work, the transition wasn't hard—but it wasn't immediate either. I had to recalibrate. Waking up was a challenge. I'd been used to early mornings and set multiple alarms just to stay on schedule. Getting back to my patients, many of whom were older and dealing with chronic illnesses, required a mental shift. The cases were complex again. There were new protocols. The electronic medical records had been updated. Even the hospital layout had changed. My favorite spot to do notes was gone—lost in renovations.

But there were care packages waiting for me, and warm welcomes from colleagues. I saw new faces and some familiar ones. The rhythm of civilian medicine eventually came back.

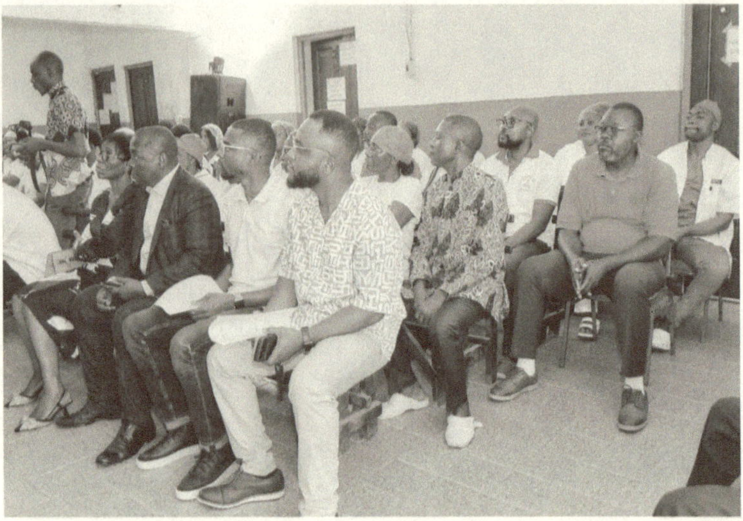

A moment of profound significance, where generosity meets urgent need. This image captures a ceremony at New-Bell Protestant Hospital, where dedicated medical staff gathered to receive vital medical supply donations. It's a powerful testament to the collaborative spirit of healing and the far-reaching impact of channeling essential resources to those who need them most. This act of kindness sparks a wave of positive change, providing hope and healing in communities that rely on such vital support.

Outside of work, home life also required adjusting. We had just moved into a new house. I had new neighbors to meet and reintroduce myself to. These were the little things—the ordinary things—that brought me joy. Mowing a lawn. Sharing a meal. Listening to the wind.

Deployment had changed me. It taught me how much we take for granted here. Our resources, our infrastructure, even our sense of safety. In Iraq, I saw how much the rest of the world looks to us—to American leadership, to American medicine, to American might.

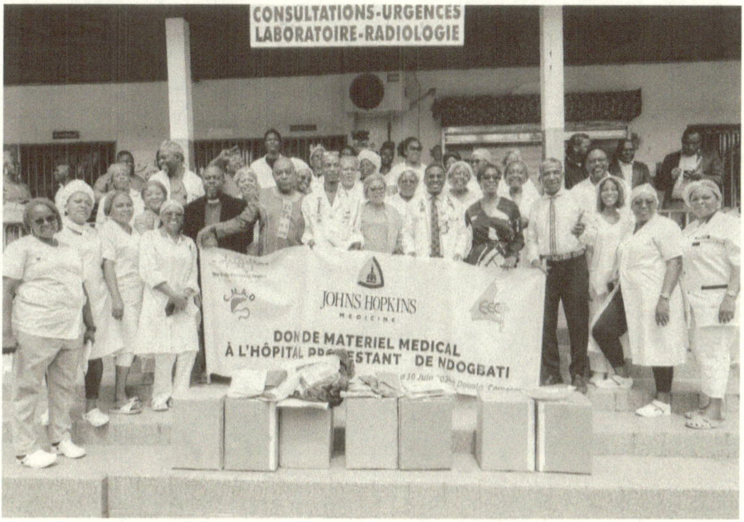

A testament to the power of generosity and its far-reaching impact. This image captures a medical supply donation, a vital act of kindness that channeled essential resources to those in need. It's a reminder that even a single contribution can spark a wave of positive change, providing hope and healing in communities that need it most.

When we held joint exercises with coalition forces—British, German, French, Estonian—there was an unspoken expectation that we, the Americans, would lead. Even during trauma activations, the other medical teams waited for our cues. They wanted to know our protocols, our placement, our procedures. I was often asked to lead the code or direct patient care. They weren't stepping back out of deference.

They were stepping back because they genuinely believed in our expertise.

That trust was humbling.

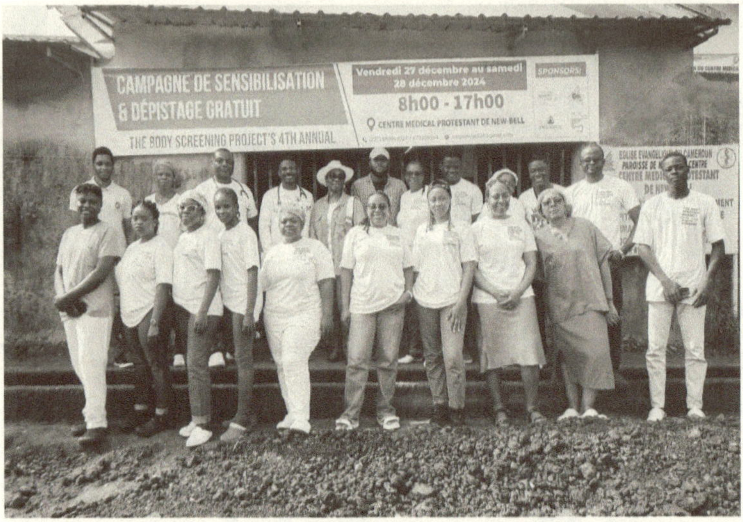
CAMPAGNE DE SENSIBILISATION
& DÉPISTAGE GRATUIT
THE BODY SCREENING PROJECT'S 4TH ANNUAL
Vendredi 27 décembre au samedi
28 décembre 2024
8h00 - 17h00
CENTRE MEDICAL PROTESTANT DE NEW-BELL
SPONSORS:

Making a tangible difference, one life at a time. The dedicated team behind The Body Screening Project's 4th Annual Health Screening in Douala, Cameroon. Together, nurses, medical assistants, and doctors provided free medical care to nearly 200 patients, a testament to the power of collective action and the profound impact of accessible healthcare. This image celebrates the spirit of humanitarianism and the unwavering commitment to serving underserved communities.

Even outside of medicine, the leadership dynamic held true. The Iraqi locals we worked with were kind, supportive, and often expressed gratitude for our presence. I gave one of them a small American flag, and the joy on his face was unforgettable. Despite the dangers, many Iraqis wanted us there. They saw our mission—defeating ISIS, restoring order—as their mission too.

The collaboration I experienced within the hospital was unlike anything I'd seen. Nurses, medics, logisticians, and support personnel all came together in ways that inspired me. It was true teamwork—fluid, responsive, and mission-focused.

And that changed how I see medicine. My time overseas made me more understanding, more compassionate. I now listen to my underserved patients with deeper empathy. Some of them, while never having served in the military, have endured hardships far greater than I did on deployment. Poverty, neglect, trauma—they've lived with so little, for so long. And now, when I care for them, I feel a renewed connection, because I understand the toll of scarcity. I understand what it means to live without.

This experience also sharpened my leadership instincts. I've become more confident in taking initiative—not just in clinical care, but in advocating for my patients, for my teams.

I believe every military member should experience deployment—not necessarily to a combat zone, but somewhere that stretches them. It builds resilience, sharpens character, and teaches you how your mind and body adapt under stress.

This deployment cemented my commitment to military medicine. I'm an attending physician now, and I plan to stay in the Army Reserve. It allows me to serve both worlds—to care for civilians and support the readiness of our armed forces. My mission is to ensure that if a soldier is hurt, I can help them heal and return home to their family. That, to me, is the heart of service.

To any reader of this story: find your purpose. Reflect on your path. It doesn't have to be medicine. It doesn't even have to be military. It could be advocacy, education, social justice, mental health—anything. But find it. Own it. And walk that road.

If my journey inspires even one person to serve in their own way, then sharing it has been worth it.

ABOUT THE AUTHOR

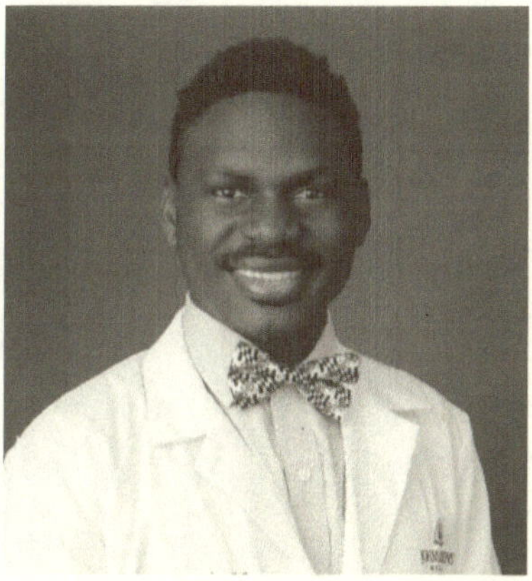

Emmanuel Dimitri Foko Tito, DO, also known as Dimitri Tito, is a military physician, author, and founder of *The Body Screening Project*. He earned his undergraduate degree in Biomedical Engineering from the University of Maryland, College Park, and went on to receive his medical degree from the West Virginia School of Osteopathic Medicine. Dr. Tito completed his Internal Medicine residency in academic medicine at Western Michigan University Homer Stryker M.D. School of Medicine and pursued additional training in Health Policy. In recognition of his dedication to public service, he was honored with the U.S. Public Health Service Excellence in Public Health Award in 2020.

Currently, Dr. Tito serves as a captain in the U.S. Army Medical Department, assigned to a Medical Readiness Operational Unit. During his military service, he has deployed to Iraq as a combat physician, where he provided critical medical care under challenging conditions. This experience not only honed his medical skills but also deepened his commitment to serving underserved populations.

www.ingramcontent.com/pod-product-compliance
Lightning Source LLC
LaVergne TN
LVHW090409210926
848480LV00002B/503
* 9 7 9 8 2 3 2 8 5 2 4 6 7 *